Study Guide to
INTRODUCTORY
PSYCHIATRY

A Companion to the
Introductory Textbook of Psychiatry,
Sixth Edition

Study Guide to
INTRODUCTORY
PSYCHIATRY

A Companion to the
Introductory Textbook of Psychiatry,
Sixth Edition

Donald W. Black, M.D.

Professor, Director of Residency Training, and
Vice Chair for Education, Department of Psychiatry,
University of Iowa Roy J. and
Lucille A. Carver College of Medicine, Iowa City, Iowa

Jordan Cates, M.D.

Private Practice of Psychiatry, Burlington, Iowa

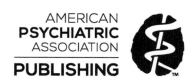

AMERICAN
PSYCHIATRIC
ASSOCIATION
PUBLISHING

If you wish to buy 50 or more copies of the same title, please go to www.appi.org/specialdiscounts for more information.

Manufactured in the United States of America on acid-free paper
20 19 18 17 16   5 4 3 2 1
First Edition

American Psychiatric Association Publishing
1000 Wilson Boulevard
Arlington, VA 22209-3901
www.appi.org

CONTENTS

PART II: ANSWER GUIDE

Foreword

As most medical students have realized by now, studying as a pre-med student in college and studying in medical school are usually very different things. Pre-med students, like most undergraduates, "cram" for examinations with the goal of getting a good grade on the exam. Most of them don't care all that much about being able to remember the material in detail at some time in the future. In the language of cognitive science, they employ "shallow encoding," while they would need to do "deep encoding" to retain and recall the information at a later time (e.g., in 5 or 10 years).

In medical school and residency, on the other hand, achieving deep encoding of learned materials is essential. You are acquiring a treasure chest of knowledge that you will use for many years to come. A good physician is a person who has preserved masses of information on diverse topics and can organize and recall them when working with any patient who walks into his or her office. A primary care physician has perhaps the greatest challenge, because of the need to diagnose and treat a diversity of diseases ranging from gastrointestinal to psychiatric. (And a large number of the problems that primary care physicians confront are psychiatric.) As one of my physician friends once said to me, "I can't be a primary care doctor because I'm not smart enough." There is a lot of truth in that statement—primary care doctors need to know **a lot.** But other specialties—cardiology, orthopedics, pediatrics—will also be called on to have good access not only to specialty knowledge but also to more general medical knowledge. You have to be "smart" to be any kind of physician.

So what is the secret of achieving deep encoding? There are in fact many. Using this study guide will facilitate some of them. One secret is to go beyond rote memorization of information to accessing it and using it to answer questions. Another is to see how knowing a piece of information is consolidated when it is approached from several different directions—for example, diagnosis, treatment planning, and understanding disease mechanisms. This study guide will facilitate those examples and many more.

We owe a lot to my colleague and coauthor of the *Introductory Textbook of Psychiatry,* and also to his coauthor of this book, for taking the time to write this study guide. They have taken painstaking care in thinking through the questions that students can answer after reading the various chapters of the textbook. When students answer a question correctly, it will help to consolidate their knowledge. When they miss a question, it will also help to consolidate, since they will need to figure out why they "got it wrong." Understanding and rectifying ignorance is as important as taking pride in having learned something well.

Donald Black has been a leader in psychiatric education for many years. He has run our residency program at Iowa with great success. He loves to teach and mentor students. He loves to see how residents can finish their training and go on to next steps—to private practice, to practice within a medical school, to a postdoctoral fellowship in clinical care (e.g., geriatrics) or in a research environment (e.g., genetics and genomics, neuroimaging). He was fortunate to have had a highly talented resident, Jordan Cates (now in private practice), help to create this wonderful study guide. Thank you, Don and Jordan!

Nancy C. Andreasen, M.D., Ph.D.
Andrew H. Woods Chair of Psychiatry and
Director, Iowa Neuroimaging Consortium,
University of Iowa Carver College of Medicine

Preface

Medical students, residents in psychiatry, and other learners have been enthusiastic about the *Introductory Textbook of Psychiatry* since it was first published in 1991. Now in its sixth edition (the DSM-5 edition), the book has changed and evolved where needed in order to stay current. After being urged to do so for many years, we have at last put together a companion study guide. This guide will give learners an opportunity to test their command of the knowledge of the material in the textbook. The questions have been written to provide emphasis and clarity to the major clinical issues described in the textbook.

We encourage readers to first answer the questions at the conclusion of each chapter in *Introductory Textbook of Psychiatry*, Sixth Edition, and then to use this study guide for additional and more detailed questions. The format replicates what might be encountered in specialty-certifying exams. Each question is followed by multiple choice responses, including plausible "distractors." The answer is then provided, with an explanation of the correct response as well as an explanation why the other answers are incorrect. Each question is linked to a page or pages in the textbook.

We believe this guide has the potential to help readers gain a much greater understanding of the material. We hope you will find this study guide interesting and useful.

Although the guide and the many questions have been reviewed many times, it is possible that an incorrect response is included. If so, please feel free to contact the senior author at donald-black@uiowa.edu.

Good luck with your studies.

Donald W. Black, M.D.
Jordan Cates, M.D.

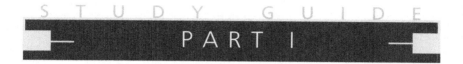

STUDY GUIDE

PART I

QUESTIONS

CHAPTER 1

Diagnosis and Classification

1.1 Which of the following terms is used to describe collections of symptoms that tend to co-occur and appear to have a characteristic course and outcome?

A. Disease.
B. Symptomatology.
C. Syndrome.
D. Pathophysiology.
E. Illness.

1.2 Which of the following is *not* a clinical reason to diagnose patients?

A. To reduce the complexity of clinical phenomena.
B. To provide the patient a label with which to identify.
C. To facilitate communication between clinicians.
D. To predict the course of illness.
E. To determine treatment options.

1.3 Which was the first edition of DSM to provide specific diagnostic criteria for mental disorders?

A. DSM-I.
B. DSM-II.
C. DSM-III.
D. DSM-IV.
E. DSM-5.

1.4   Which of the following is *not* an advantage of the DSM system?

   A. It has substantially improved reliability of diagnoses.
   B. It has substantially improved validity of diagnoses.
   C. It has clarified the diagnostic process and history taking.
   D. It has clarified and facilitated the process of differential diagnosis.
   E. All of the above are advantages of the DSM system.

1.5   You are asked to evaluate a 55-year-old man on a general medical floor. You determine that he is delirious because of a hepatic encephalopathy. You learn that he drinks large quantities of distilled spirits daily and smokes one pack of cigarettes per day. Taking into account the International Classification of Diseases (ICD) and DSM rules, how would you record his diagnoses (i.e., in order of importance)?

   A. Delirium (principal diagnosis), alcohol use disorder, tobacco use disorder.
   B. Delirium due to hepatic encephalopathy (principal diagnosis), alcohol use disorder, tobacco use disorder.
   C. Alcohol use disorder (provisional diagnosis), delirium due to hepatic encephalopathy, tobacco use disorder.
   D. Hepatic encephalopathy, delirium due to hepatic encephalopathy (principal diagnosis), alcohol use disorder, tobacco use disorder.
   E. Delirium due to hepatic encephalopathy, hepatic encephalopathy, alcohol use disorder, tobacco use disorder.

1.6   You are evaluating a patient in the emergency room who you believe is likely experiencing a psychotic manic episode (bipolar I disorder with psychotic features). The patient is a poor historian, and you are not currently able to obtain collateral information to confirm the diagnosis. According to DSM, how should you document the diagnosis to reflect your uncertainty?

   A. Rule out bipolar disorder, type 1.
   B. Evaluate for bipolar disorder, type 1.
   C. Bipolar disorder, type 1, versus psychosis not otherwise specified.
   D. Bipolar disorder, type 1 (provisional).
   E. Bipolar disorder, type 1.

1.7　You are seeing 25-year-old woman in the outpatient clinic for a routine follow-up visit. Her major problems reported at the visit are her stormy interpersonal relationships and frequent anger outbursts. You conclude that these symptoms result from her borderline personality disorder. The patient's symptoms also meet criteria for generalized anxiety disorder, and she smokes 10 cigarettes daily. How would you record the diagnoses according to DSM-5?

A. Axis I: generalized anxiety disorder, tobacco use disorder; Axis II: borderline personality disorder (principal diagnosis).
B. Borderline personality disorder (principal diagnosis), generalized anxiety disorder, tobacco use disorder.
C. Generalized anxiety disorder, borderline personality disorder, tobacco use disorder.
D. Tobacco use disorder, borderline personality disorder, generalized anxiety disorder.
E. Borderline personality disorder (provisional), generalized anxiety disorder, tobacco use disorder.

CHAPTER 2

Interviewing and Assessment

2.1 A psychiatrist asks a patient to recall a list of three objects ("orange, airplane, tobacco") after 5 minutes. What type of memory does this test?

   A. Ultrashort-term memory.
   B. Very short-term memory.
   C. Short-term memory.
   D. Medium-term memory.
   E. Long-term memory.

2.2 A psychiatrist asks a patient to tell her what the phrase "don't cry over spilled milk" means. The patient replies, "Milk isn't worth crying over because it's easy to come by." What does the patient's answer suggest?

   A. Illogicality.
   B. Poor abstraction.
   C. Derailment.
   D. Circumstantiality.
   E. Poverty of content of speech.

2.3 A man believes he is preventing cancer and maximizing his health by taking an expensive but otherwise innocuous herbal supplement. If asked, he will discuss the supplement with great interest but dismisses evidence that does not confirm his beliefs. Otherwise, this interest in the supplement has no significant influence on his day-to-day life. Which of the following terms best describes the man's beliefs?

A. Overvalued ideation.
B. Delusion.
C. Poor abstraction.
D. Impaired fund of knowledge.
E. Illogicality.

2.4   A patient admits to her psychiatrist that she sometimes worries that events she reads about in magazines indirectly comment on her personal life. For example, one of her favorite magazines had a recipe for banana cream pie, which made her think that somehow the editor knew this was her favorite pie. The psychiatrist asks her if she really believes this, and the patient reports that sometimes it does seem "silly." What term best describes the woman's suspicion?

A. Illogicality.
B. Persecutory delusions.
C. Delusions of reference.
D. Ideas of reference.
E. Thought broadcasting.

2.5   A 35-year-old woman reports to her psychiatrist that, as part of a government conspiracy, a mind control device was implanted in her brain. She believes the FBI (or possibly the CIA) is using this device to spy on her. Further, she says the device can control her body movements, making her feel like a puppet on a string. She describes how the device can remove thoughts from her brain like a vacuum cleaner while implanting thoughts that are not hers. Which of the following symptoms is *not* consistent with this patient's delusional system?

A. Delusions of passivity.
B. Thought withdrawal.
C. Thought insertion.
D. Somatic delusions.
E. Persecutory delusions.

2.6   A psychiatrist asks a patient where she lives. She replies, "I live in Springfield. It will be spring in another couple of months, but at least this winter has been mild. The winter tends to be pretty bad in Atlanta, which is where I lived until I moved to Springfield, but birds fly south in the winter. I'd really like to go to the beach just now." What is this an example of?

A. Tangentiality.
B. Circumstantiality.
C. Incoherence.
D. Illogicality.
E. Derailment.

2.7 A psychiatrist asks a patient if he enjoyed his own birthday party the prior week. The patient responds by laboriously describing preparations for the party and then going into minute detail about the party, including such minutiae as the order of arrival of the guests and vivid descriptions of the appetizers. Ten minutes into this story, the psychiatrist realizes that the patient never answered his question. What is this an example of?

A. Circumstantiality.
B. Pressured speech.
C. Derailment.
D. Tangentiality.
E. Distractible speech.

2.8 Which of the following options is a pattern of speech in which sounds rather than meaningful relationships among words appears to govern word choice?

A. Incoherence.
B. Clanging.
C. Distractible speech.
D. Pressured speech.
E. Alogia.

2.9 A psychiatrist is interviewing a manic patient. The patient speaks very rapidly, and it is very difficult for the psychiatrist to get a word in. The patient is unable to adequately answer many routine questions because he is distracted by objects in the room such as chairs, the psychiatrist's neck tie, and the clock on the wall. Which of the following options best describes the patient's speech?

A. Pressured speech.
B. Distractible speech.
C. Both pressured speech and distracted speech.
D. Catatonic excitement.
E. Circumstantiality.

2.10 In response to a routine question, a patient begins to answer appropriately, but stops talking mid-sentence, and stares off into space for 15 seconds. She then asks the interviewer to repeat the question. What does this exemplify?

A. Poverty of speech.
B. Poverty of content of speech.
C. Circumstantiality.
D. Perseveration.
E. Thought blocking.

2.11 A psychiatrist notes that a patient is very slow to answer questions and that his speech and body movements are slow. What is the correct term for this symptom?

A. Depression.
B. Psychomotor retardation.
C. Psychomotor agitation.
D. Thought blocking.
E. Alogia.

— CHAPTER 3 —

Neurobiology and Genetics of Mental Illness

3.1 Which of the following is *not* a primary function of the prefrontal system?

A. High-order abstract thought.
B. Creative problem solving.
C. Fear processing.
D. Temporal sequencing of behavior.
E. Moral judgment.

3.2 Which of the following areas of the brain have a high concentration of dopamine D_2 receptors and may be important sites for antipsychotic drug action?

A. Locus coeruleus.
B. Caudate and putamen.
C. Raphe nuclei.
D. Nucleus basalis.
E. None of the above.

3.3 Which part of the brain is dedicated to speech production?

A. Broca's area.
B. Nucleus basalis.
C. Angular gyrus.
D. Wernicke's area.
E. Amygdala.

3.4 The nucleus accumbens is a key part of which functional system in the brain?

A. Executive system.
B. Limbic system.
C. Memory system.
D. Attention system.
E. Reward system.

3.5 What is the primary neurotransmitter in the brain reward system, which is also associated with adventuresome and exploratory behaviors?

A. Dopamine.
B. Norepinephrine.
C. γ-Aminobutyric acid (GABA).
D. Serotonin.
E. Glutamate.

3.6 Where does the brain's norepinephrine system originate?

A. Raphe nuclei.
B. Hypothalamus.
C. Ventral tegmental area.
D. Locus coeruleus.
E. Nucleus accumbens.

3.7 Which of the following nuclei in the brain contains the cell bodies of an important group of acetylcholine neurons?

A. Nucleus basalis.
B. Locus coeruleus.
C. Raphe nuclei.
D. Substantia nigra.
E. Caudate nucleus.

3.8 Which neurotransmitter provides inhibitory modulation to the globus pallidus, which if lost, will result in the choreiform movements of Huntington's disease?

A. Dopamine.
B. Serotonin.

C. Acetylcholine.

D. Glutamate.

E. GABA.

3.9 Family studies of mental illness have shown that most major mental illnesses "run in families." Which of the following is *not* an essential element of a family study?

    A. Identifying people with the disorder of interest (e.g., schizophrenia).

    B. Identifying people who can serve as control subjects.

    C. Interviewing first-degree relatives of ill persons and control subjects.

    D. Comparing rates of the disorder of interest in relatives of those with the mental illness in question and relatives of control subjects.

    E. Showing that the illness in question is inherited.

3.10 Which type of study applies statistical analyses to large databases containing DNA from thousands of individuals affected by specific disorders?

    A. Linkage study.

    B. Candidate gene study.

    C. Genome-wide association study.

    D. Copy number variant survey.

    E. Microarray analysis.

━ CHAPTER 4 ━

Neurodevelopmental (Child) Disorders

4.1   What is the standard test used to assess the intelligence of children between 6 and 16 years of age?

A. Stanford-Binet Intelligence Scale.
B. Wechsler Intelligence Scale for Children (WISC).
C. Peabody Picture Vocabulary Test.
D. Kaufman ABC.
E. Wechsler Preschool and Primary Scale of Intelligence.

4.2   What is the standard deviation of IQ on the WISC-IV?

A. 100.
B. 85.
C. 15.
D. 25.
E. 115.

4.3   Which of the following scales can be used to assess for attention-deficit/hyperactivity disorder (ADHD)?

A. Benton Visual Retention Test.
B. Vineland Adaptive Behavior Scale.
C. Thematic Apperception Test.
D. Conners Teacher Rating Scale—Revised.
E. Bender-Gestalt.

4.4   What is the most common heritable cause of intellectual disability?

   A. Down syndrome.
   B. Fragile X.
   C. Tay-Sachs.
   D. Prader-Willi syndrome.
   E. Williams syndrome.

4.5   A 25-year-old man with intellectual disability has lived in a
       group home all of his adult life. He can read his name and a few
       other words. He is able to take care of his activities of daily living
       such as bathing and other personal hygiene tasks and doing
       laundry. He was in special education classes throughout school.
       What is the probable severity of his intellectual disability?

   A. Mild.
   B. Moderate.
   C. Severe.
   D. Profound.
   E. Unable to estimate.

4.6   What is the DSM-5 diagnosis for a child who stutters?

   A. Language disorder.
   B. Speech sound disorder.
   C. Childhood-onset fluency disorder.
   D. Social (pragmatic) communication disorder.
   E. Autism spectrum disorder.

4.7   An 8-year-old boy is brought to a child psychiatrist for an evalu-
       ation. His parents report that he is socially awkward and has
       trouble making friends. His grades are very good. The boy is po-
       lite but overly formal in conversation. He avoids eye contact. His
       parents report that he sticks to a rigid routine at home and has an
       unusually intense interest in U.S. presidents and can name all of
       them in correct order. When this is brought up, the child begins a
       lengthy discourse on them. What is the best diagnosis?

   A. Language disorder.
   B. Speech sound disorder.
   C. Childhood-onset fluency disorder.

D. Social (pragmatic) communication disorder.

E. Autism spectrum disorder.

4.8   How does treatment with stimulant medications affect risk of substance abuse in persons diagnosed with ADHD?

A. Use of stimulant medications increases the risk of any substance abuse.

B. Use of stimulant medications decreases the risk of any substance abuse.

C. Use of stimulant medications does not affect the risk of substance abuse.

D. Use of stimulant medications is associated with a worse long-term outcome.

E. Use of stimulant medications increases the risk for abuse of stimulant medications only.

4.9   What is the prevalence of ADHD in children?

A. 1%–2%.

B. 5%.

C. 10%.

D. 20%.

E. >30%.

4.10   A 9-year-old boy is brought to his pediatrician by his parents, who are concerned about the possibility of ADHD. A written report from his teacher says that he is frequently in trouble for fighting with other children and that he refuses to obey classroom rules. He frequently steals small items from his peers and the school cafeteria. He also talks out of turn and has trouble staying in his seat. His parents report that he has lots of energy and that he "bounces off the walls" at home. He talks back to his parents. Which of the following symptoms in this case is suggestive of ADHD?

A. Fighting with other children.

B. Refusal to obey classroom rules.

C. Stealing.

D. Talking back to parents.

E. Difficulty staying in his seat.

4.11 Which of the following medications is a first-line treatment for ADHD?

A. Guanfacine.
B. Methylphenidate.
C. Clonidine.
D. Bupropion.
E. Atomoxetine.

4.12 Which of the following is *not* a common side effect of the stimulant medications commonly used to treat ADHD?

A. Weight gain.
B. Insomnia.
C. Stomach upset.
D. Irritability.
E. Appetite suppression.

4.13 A 9-year-old boy of average intelligence is making satisfactory grades in all subjects in school with the exception of math, which he is failing. His Iowa Test of Basic Skills score confirms satisfactory performance on all subjects except math, which is considerably lower than average. He sometimes shows irritation and frustration in the classroom during math class, but his behavior is otherwise unremarkable. His parents do not have concerns about his mood or behavior at home. What is the most beneficial intervention for this child?

A. Remedial instruction in math and instruction in compensatory learning strategies.
B. Start methylphenidate.
C. Start fluoxetine.
D. Start atomoxetine.
E. Referral for cognitive-behavioral therapy.

4.14 Which of the following is *not* considered a stereotypic movement when considering the diagnosis of stereotypic movement disorder?

A. Head banging.
B. Rocking.
C. Hitting one's own body.

D. Nonrhythmic, jerky movements of the neck.

E. Hand waving.

4.15 How is the diagnosis of Tourette's disorder different from a persistent motor or vocal tic disorder?

A. Patients with Tourette's disorder have coprolalia (offensive vocal tics).

B. Tics in Tourette's disorder are of longer duration than tics that occur in motor or vocal tic disorder.

C. Patients with Tourette's disorder have both motor and vocal tics.

D. Tourette's disorder is associated with streptococcal infection.

E. Tourette's disorder has high comorbidity with obsessive-compulsive disorder.

4.16 Which of the following medications are U.S. Food and Drug Administration (FDA) approved for treatment of pediatric depression?

A. Fluoxetine and escitalopram.

B. Citalopram and paroxetine.

C. Venlafaxine and nefazodone.

D. Sertraline and citalopram.

E. Escitalopram and citalopram.

— CHAPTER 5 —

Schizophrenia Spectrum and Other Psychotic Disorders

5.1   Which of the following statements *mischaracterizes* schizophrenia?

     A. Patients have a "split" personality.
     B. Patients have disability in their capacity to think clearly.
     C. Patients have disability in their capacity to experience normal emotions.
     D. Patients typically develop symptoms in early adulthood.
     E. Patients often develop bizarre hallucinations and delusions.

5.2   You have been seeing a 45-year-old man in the outpatient clinic for "stress." He relates his stress to what he believes was a conspiracy by former coworkers to get him fired from his previous job by "arranging" work-related incidents that would reflect poorly on him. He has threatened to sue, but because of lack of evidence, no lawyer has agreed to take his case. As his psychiatrist, you find yourself unable to get him to talk about other issues. He has never had hallucinations, disorganized behavior, mania, or frank depression. What is the most likely diagnosis?

     A. Schizophrenia.
     B. Schizoaffective disorder.
     C. Schizophreniform disorder.
     D. Delusional disorder.
     E. Bipolar I disorder.

5.3 At what age do women typically develop schizophrenia?

A. 13–18 years.
B. 18–25 years.
C. 21–30 years.
D. 35–50 years.
E. >50 years.

5.4 Which of the following is an example of a "first-rank" symptom of schizophrenia as identified by psychiatrist Kurt Schneider?

A. The patient believes thoughts are being inserted into his or her mind.
B. The patient believes the government is spying on him or her.
C. The patient believes that his or her masturbation has led to insanity.
D. The patient believes the somatic delusion that his or her heart has stopped beating.
E. The patient experiences the tactile hallucination that insects are crawling under his or her skin.

5.5 You are evaluating a 30-year-old woman with schizophrenia on a psychiatric inpatient unit. She reports that she has died and has gone to heaven to be with Jesus. She will not accept any evidence to the contrary. What type of delusion is this?

A. Persecutory delusion.
B. Grandiose delusion.
C. Nihilistic delusion.
D. Somatic delusion.
E. Religious delusion.

5.6 Which phase of schizophrenia is characterized by subtle behavior changes that include social withdrawal, work impairment, blunting of emotion, avolition, and odd ideas and behavior?

A. Prodromal phase.
B. Active phase.
C. Residual phase.
D. Cataleptic phase.
E. Schizoaffective phase.

5.7   You are treating a patient with schizophrenia on an inpatient unit. The patient has displayed disorganized behavior throughout hospitalization. One day at morning rounds, the patient mimics your hand gestures without reason. What is the term for this behavior?

A. Echolalia.
B. Echopraxia.
C. Catalepsy.
D. Negativism.
E. Stereotypy.

5.8   A 20-year-old man with schizophrenia comes to your clinic for a scheduled follow-up visit, accompanied by his mother, with whom he lives. His disorder is well controlled with low-dose antipsychotic medication. He reports mild auditory hallucinations but says they do not bother him. His mother is concerned that the patient is inactive much of the day and must be prompted to groom himself. He prefers to watch TV all day without engaging in any other activities. The patient shows some affective blunting but denies depressed mood. He reports restful sleep and has a healthy appetite. He tolerates his medication without noticeable adverse effects and says he feels "pretty good" about his current situation. How should you address the mother's concerns?

A. Prescribe a stimulant to increase his energy.
B. Prescribe an antidepressant to treat his negative symptoms.
C. Reassess the patient for schizoaffective disorder and consider adding a mood stabilizer.
D. Reduce the dose of the antipsychotic medication.
E. Provide psychoeducation to the patient's mother.

5.9   A 24-year-old woman is admitted to an inpatient psychiatric unit for acute psychosis. She endorses auditory hallucinations and persecutory delusions and has an inappropriate affect. She has no previous episodes, she has not been abusing substances, and medical workup does not show a clear etiology for her symptoms. She has not shown clear symptoms of major depression or of mania. At this point, her total duration of illness is 2 weeks. What is the best diagnosis at this time?

A. Schizophrenia.
B. Schizoaffective disorder.
C. Schizophreniform disorder.
D. Brief psychotic disorder.
E. Bipolar disorder.

5.10 Postpartum psychosis is a subtype of which DSM-5 psychotic disorder?

A. Schizophrenia.
B. Schizoaffective disorder.
C. Schizophreniform disorder.
D. Brief psychotic disorder.
E. Bipolar disorder.

5.11 A 24-year-old woman is admitted to an inpatient psychiatric unit for acute psychosis in the setting of medication noncompliance. She reports auditory hallucinations and persecutory delusions and has an inappropriate affect. She has no previous episodes, she has not been abusing substances, and medical workup does not show a clear etiology of her symptoms. She has not shown clear symptoms of major depression or of mania. This episode has been going on for the past 2 weeks. Two months previously, she had her first psychotic episode, which lasted for 3 weeks, but she went into remission with antipsychotic therapy. What is the best diagnosis?

A. Schizophrenia.
B. Schizoaffective disorder.
C. Schizophreniform disorder.
D. Brief psychotic disorder.
E. Bipolar disorder.

5.12 Which of the following risk factors is associated with poor outcome in schizophrenia?

A. Female sex.
B. Insidious onset of symptoms.
C. Short prodrome.
D. Currently married.
E. Late onset.

5.13 Which of the following individuals has the *lowest* risk for developing schizophrenia?

A. Sibling of a person with schizophrenia.
B. Child of parents each having schizophrenia.
C. Identical twin of a person with schizophrenia.
D. Person having a sibling with schizophrenia and one parent with schizophrenia.
E. Child with one parent with schizophrenia.

5.14 Which of the following vulnerability genes associated with schizophrenia has a known direct effect on dopamine production?

A. Catechol-O-methyltransferase *(COMT)*.
B. Neuregulin 1 *(NRG1)*.
C. D-Amino acid oxidase activator *(DAOA)*.
D. Metabotropic glutamate receptor 3 *(GRM3)*.
E. None of the above.

5.15 Which of the following brain abnormalities in schizophrenia is associated with poor premorbid functioning, negative symptoms, poor response to treatment, and cognitive impairment?

A. Sulcal enlargement.
B. Cerebellar atrophy.
C. Decreased size of frontal lobe.
D. Ventricular enlargement.
E. Decreased size of thalamus.

5.16 Which of the following mechanisms of action has been hypothesized to explain the effectiveness of antipsychotic drugs?

A. Dopamine (D_2) receptor blockade.
B. 5-Hydroxytryptamine (serotonin) type 2 receptor ($5\text{-}HT_2$) blockade.
C. Glutamate receptor blockade.
D. Inhibition of serotonin reuptake.
E. Inhibition of dopamine reuptake.

5.17 Which of the following psychosocial treatments is known to reduce rates of relapse in schizophrenia?

A. Cognitive-behavioral therapy.
B. Interpersonal psychotherapy.
C. Social skills training.
D. Family therapy.
E. Vocational rehabilitation.

5.18 Which of the following features is consistent with a diagnosis of
schizoaffective disorder but not major depression or bipolar disorder?

A. Manic episodes accompanied by hallucinations and delusions.
B. Depressive episodes accompanied by hallucinations and delusions.
C. Hallucinations and delusions for at least 2 weeks in the absence of a major mood episode.
D. Presence of a mixed mood episode accompanied by hallucinations and delusions.
E. Symptoms of a major mood episode present for 25% of the total duration of the illness.

— CHAPTER 6 —

Mood Disorders

6.1 Who first differentiated bipolar disorder from schizophrenia?

A. Eugen Bleuler.
B. Emil Kraepelin.
C. Sigmund Freud.
D. Kurt Schneider.
E. Carl Jung.

6.2 Bipolar II disorder first appeared in which edition of the DSM?

A. DSM-I.
B. DSM-II.
C. DSM-III.
D. DSM-IV.
E. DSM-5.

6.3 What is the minimum duration of a manic episode?

A. 12 hours.
B. 1–2 days.
C. 4 days.
D. 7 days.
E. 2 weeks.

6.4 Which of the following features is consistent with a hypomanic episode but *not* a manic episode?

A. Presence of psychotic symptoms such as hallucinations and delusions.
B. Duration of at least 1 week.

C. Elevated mood.

D. Decreased need for sleep.

E. Lack of marked social and occupational dysfunction.

6.5 A 28-year-old man is brought to the emergency room by the police for a psychiatric evaluation after his neighbors reported that he was behaving erratically. He is irritable and displays pressured speech, and he has only slept a few hours in the past several days. He believes the FBI has implanted a microchip in his brain to record his thoughts and send him messages. He has been spending several hours each day making blueprints for lethal booby traps for his home to protect himself against government agents. He derails frequently in conversation. His physical examination is significant for dental caries, and his urine drug screen is positive for amphetamines. Why would it be premature to diagnose this patient with bipolar I disorder based on this presentation?

A. Presence of psychosis.

B. Persecutory delusions.

C. Mood is irritable rather than elevated.

D. Amphetamines present in drug screen.

E. Lack of grandiosity.

6.6 Which of the following features is more characteristic of bipolar II disorder than bipolar I disorder?

A. Multiple hospitalizations.

B. Depressive episodes more prominent during the course of illness.

C. Presence of psychotic symptoms.

D. Lack of a comorbid substance use disorder.

E. Better response to lithium.

6.7 A 10-year-old boy is brought to his family physician by his parents. He has had recurrent severe behavioral outbursts at home and at school several times a week for the past several years. Outbursts are typically in reaction to minor disappointments or when he is asked to do routine chores. His parents did not seek attention for this problem because they thought he would outgrow it. Between outbursts, the boy's mood is "grumpy." What is the most likely diagnosis?

A. Disruptive mood dysregulation disorder.
B. Bipolar II disorder.
C. Major depressive disorder.
D. Persistent depressive disorder.
E. Unspecified depressive disorder.

6.8   A 35-year-old woman comes to your clinic to establish care. She reports that she has been depressed since adolescence with ongoing symptoms of low mood throughout the day, feelings of worthlessness, hypersomnia, low energy, and poor concentration. She does not remember any recent period in the past several years that she was free of depression. What is the best diagnosis?

A. Major depressive disorder.
B. Persistent depressive disorder.
C. Disruptive mood dysregulation disorder.
D. Unspecified depressive disorder.
E. Bipolar II disorder.

6.9   A 30-year-old man comes to your clinic seeking help for depression. He has been feeling depressed most of the day for the past 3 weeks. He complains of restless sleep, low energy, poor concentration, and decreased appetite. He has lost interest in his work, and he spends most of his time watching TV, although with poor attention. He has lost 5 lbs. since this episode started. He has had thoughts of wanting to hang himself, but he does not think he would actually try to kill himself because of his family. This is his fourth episode of depression since adolescence. Prior episodes have resolved spontaneously within a few months, and he is symptom free between episodes. What is the best diagnosis?

A. Disruptive mood dysregulation disorder.
B. Bipolar I disorder.
C. Major depressive disorder.
D. Persistent depressive disorder.
E. Unspecified depressive disorder.

6.10   A 60-year-old woman develops depressive symptoms following the death of her husband. She has trouble sleeping, feelings of guilt, low energy, decreased appetite, and difficulty paying attention in conversations. She has not had a prior episode of depression, and she is not suicidal. Her symptoms have been ongoing for 3 weeks. What is the best diagnosis?

A. Bereavement.
B. Major depressive disorder.
C. Unspecified depressive disorder.
D. Persistent depressive disorder.
E. Bipolar II disorder.

6.11 What does it mean for a patient with bipolar disorder to have "rapid cycling"?

A. Severe mood swings throughout the day.
B. Switching between mania and depression several times throughout a week.
C. At least four distinct mood episodes (mania, depression, etc.) in 1 year.
D. At least four distinct mood episodes (mania, depression, etc.) in 1 month.
E. None of the above.

6.12 A major depressive episode characterized by interpersonal rejection sensitivity, increased appetite, and hypersomnia indicates which of the following?

A. Atypical features.
B. Melancholic features.
C. Catatonic features.
D. Diurnal variation.
E. None of the above.

6.13 What is the lifetime prevalence for major depression?

A. 3%.
B. 10%.
C. 17%.
D. 38%.
E. >50%.

6.14 Which of the following medications is *least* appropriate for the treatment of acute mania?

A. Carbamazepine.
B. Lithium.
C. Second-generation antipsychotic.
D. Gabapentin.
E. Valproate.

6.15 What class of medication is the first-line treatment for depression?

A. Second-generation antipsychotic.
B. Selective serotonin reuptake inhibitor.
C. Tricyclic antidepressant.
D. Serotonin-norepinephrine reuptake inhibitor.
E. Monoamine oxidase inhibitor.

CHAPTER 7

Anxiety Disorders

7.1   A 7-year-old girl is brought to a therapist by her parents because of she refuses to attend school. She has pretended to be sick ("Mommy, my tummy hurts") several times each week for the past month to avoid going to school. She reports fear of being away from her mother during the day, and she reports nightmares of "bad accidents" happening to her mother. What is the most likely diagnosis?

     A. Generalized anxiety disorder.
     B. Social anxiety disorder.
     C. Separation anxiety disorder.
     D. Panic disorder.
     E. Specific phobia.

7.2   A teacher asks the parents of a 10-year-old boy to meet with her. She reports that since the boy started at the school 2 months ago, he has barely said a word and participates minimally in classroom activities. The parents report that, on the contrary, the boy is very talkative at home and they haven't noticed any areas of concern. What is the most likely diagnosis?

     A. Generalized anxiety disorder.
     B. Social anxiety disorder.
     C. Separation anxiety disorder.
     D. Selective mutism.
     E. Specific phobia.

7.3   What is the primary fear that underlies social anxiety disorder?

A. Social situations.
B. Intimacy.
C. Sexual inadequacy.
D. Public humiliation.
E. Narcissistic injury.

7.4   What is the typical age at onset for social anxiety disorder?

A. Preschool years.
B. Elementary school age.
C. Adolescence.
D. Early adulthood.
E. Middle adulthood.

7.5   All but which of the following medication classes is effective in treating social anxiety disorder?

A. Selective serotonin reuptake inhibitors (SSRIs).
B. Monoamine oxidase inhibitors (MAOIs).
C. Tricyclic antidepressants (TCAs).
D. β-Blockers.
E. Benzodiazepines.

7.6   A 24-year-old woman presents to the emergency room complaining of the sudden onset of shortness of breath, dizziness, diaphoresis, chest pain, and a sense of impending doom. Her medical work-up is negative, and her symptoms resolve within 30 minutes. She has had multiple prior episodes and fears her next spell. She avoids public places for fear of having an episode in public. What is the most likely diagnosis?

A. Generalized anxiety disorder.
B. Specific phobia.
C. Panic disorder.
D. Separation anxiety disorder.
E. Social anxiety disorder.

7.7 Which of the following medications is the best long-term treatment for specific phobia?

A. Fluoxetine.
B. Lorazepam.
C. Sertraline.
D. Alprazolam.
E. None of the above.

7.8 Which two psychiatric disorders are the most likely to be comorbid with panic disorder?

A. Generalized anxiety disorder and major depressive disorder.
B. Generalized anxiety disorder and social anxiety disorder.
C. Major depressive disorder and alcohol use disorder.
D. Specific phobia and alcohol use disorder.
E. Persistent depressive disorder and generalized anxiety disorder.

7.9 What substance has been implicated in the "false suffocation alarm" theory of panic disorder?

A. CO_2.
B. O_2.
C. Sodium lactate.
D. Melatonin.
E. CO.

7.10 A 20-year-old college student develops symptoms of intense anxiety, racing heart, dizziness, diaphoresis, and shortness of breath. The symptoms resolve within less than 30 minutes. Prior to developing these symptoms, he had consumed several cups of coffee in an effort to stay up late studying for an exam. He had not had prior episodes. What is the most likely diagnosis?

A. Panic disorder.
B. Specific phobia.
C. Social phobia.
D. Substance-induced anxiety disorder.
E. Generalized anxiety disorder.

7.11 What is the literal meaning of the term *agoraphobia*?

A. Fear of people.
B. Fear of crowds.
C. Fear of open spaces.
D. Fear of the marketplace.
E. Fear of enclosed spaces.

7.12 A 30-year-old woman complains to her new family physician of feeling "wound up" all the time. She describes herself as a "worrier" and feels she has always been this way, always worrying about "everything." She has chronic insomnia and reports having muscle tension in her neck and shoulders. She has a hard time concentrating. She drinks a cup of coffee in the morning but otherwise does not use stimulants. She denies depression or substance abuse. What is the most likely diagnosis?

A. Separation anxiety disorder.
B. Generalized anxiety disorder.
C. Substance-induced anxiety disorder.
D. Agoraphobia.
E. Panic disorder.

7.13 The treatment of generalized anxiety disorder usually involves individual psychotherapy in addition to which of the following medications?

A. Buspirone.
B. Escitalopram.
C. Venlafaxine.
D. Duloxetine.
E. All of the above.

— CHAPTER 8 —

Obsessive-Compulsive and Related Disorders

8.1   Which of the following is *not* considered an obsession according to DSM-5?

A. Recurrent concerns about germs or contamination.
B. Fixation on the appearance of a particular body part.
C. Intrusive and disturbing thoughts about a loved one being murdered.
D. Obsessive desire to achieve an ambitious career goal to fulfill long-standing dreams.
E. Need to collect worthless items and being unable to throw things away.

8.2   Which of the following is *not* a common compulsive ritual?

A. Handwashing.
B. Counting.
C. Gambling.
D. Checking.
E. Symmetrical arranging.

8.3   A 34-year-old man with generalized anxiety disorder tells his psychiatrist he is worried that he may have obsessive-compulsive disorder (OCD) after reading an article on the Internet. He checks his door locks repetitively each morning before leaving for work, which may take 5–10 minutes. He worries that burglars could enter the house, but he is able to put the thought out of his mind after leaving his home. He has had these behaviors since adolescence. There is no family history of OCD. On the basis of this information, what should the psychiatrist tell this patient?

A. We should start clomipramine for OCD.
B. OCD is not likely, based on the age at onset of your symptoms.
C. OCD is not likely, based on your negative family history.
D. OCD is not likely because your symptoms are so mild.
E. OCD is not likely, based on your established diagnosis of generalized anxiety disorder.

8.4   A 25-year-old man sees a psychiatrist for help for his OCD. He spends over 2–3 hours each day arranging his bookshelves at home and is fed up with his need to do this. He feels he is unable to stop his behavior and is afraid to have people over to his home for fear they might "mess up" the shelves. He has never sought treatment because he thought he could handle it on his own. Which of the following options is a reasonable treatment strategy for this patient?

A. Clomipramine.
B. Fluoxetine.
C. Behavior therapy.
D. Clomipramine and behavior therapy.
E. All of the above.

8.5   A patient comes to establish care with a new psychiatrist for treatment of OCD. He has been to several psychiatrists and therapists in the past 10 years, but he is frustrated because none of the treatments has been curative. How should the psychiatrist respond to this patient's concern?

A. Review the patient's adherence to specific medications.
B. Ask how long the patient has been able to stay in exposure therapy.
C. Recommend a new medication.
D. Inform the patient that OCD tends to be chronic.
E. None of the above.

8.6   Which of the following disorders appears to be genetically linked with OCD?

A. Pediatric autoimmune neuropsychiatric disorders associated with streptococcal infections (PANDAS).
B. Tourette's disorder.

C. Epilepsy.

D. Huntington's disease.

E. Sydenham's chorea.

8.7   A 17-year-old woman is brought to a psychiatrist because of the concerns of her parents. She spends an inordinate amount of time staring at her nose in the mirror and has been saving income from a part-time job for a rhinoplasty. The patient says her nose is ugly and that her classmates stare at it, making fun of her through coded references. She cannot be reassured by her family that her nose looks normal and is even attractive. On examination, the nose appears unremarkable. She reports feeling demoralized by her concerns about her nose but has no history of depression, and she is not psychotic. There is no evidence of a thought disorder or disorganization. What is the best diagnosis?

A. OCD with somatic obsessions.

B. Obsessive-compulsive personality disorder.

C. Delusional disorder, somatic type.

D. Body dysmorphic disorder.

E. Schizophrenia.

8.8   A 30-year-old man sees a psychiatrist at his wife's insistence. She is concerned about the possibility of him having OCD after watching a TV program about hoarding. He has an extensive video game collection that he has been accumulating since age 7. His collection is neatly arranged on shelves that do not take up much space. He is proud of his collection, and he would never think about getting rid of a single title because he sees no reason to do so. He enjoys playing video games for an hour or so each day, but otherwise keeps busy with work. He is tight with money and insists on doing many household chores himself because he believes his family can't ever do things to his standards. He has rigid political ideas that he is happy to share with others on his favorite social networking site. He does not feel that he has a significant problem with depression or anxiety. What is the most likely diagnosis?

A. OCD.

B. Obsessive-compulsive personality disorder.

C. Hoarding disorder.

D. Gaming addiction.

E. Partner relational problem.

8.9   What kind of psychotherapy is recommended for trichotillomania?

   A. Supportive psychotherapy.
   B. Behavioral therapy.
   C. Psychodynamic psychotherapy.
   D. Interpersonal psychotherapy.
   E. Acceptance and commitment therapy.

8.10   Which tricyclic antidepressant has shown benefit for trichotillo-
       mania?

   A. Imipramine.
   B. Doxepin.
   C. Clomipramine.
   D. Amitriptyline.
   E. Nortriptyline.

8.11   A 31-year old woman has many open and bleeding sores on her
       forearms. She has sought help from dermatologists, who have pre-
       scribed various creams, all to no avail. The last dermatologist in-
       sisted that the woman seek a psychiatric evaluation. What is the
       most likely diagnosis?

   A. Trichotillomania.
   B. Unspecified obsessive-compulsive and related disorder.
   C. Excoriation disorder.
   D. Delusional disorder, somatic type.
   E. OCD.

8.12   In excoriation disorder, where is the most common site for skin
       picking?

   A. Face.
   B. Hands.
   C. Feet.
   D. Arms.
   E. Torso.

— CHAPTER 9 —

Trauma- and Stressor-Related Disorders

9.1 A 7-year-old boy is brought to a child psychiatrist by his new foster parents. He had been removed from his biological parents at an early age because of neglect, and he has been in several foster homes. They report that he is sullen much of the time and almost never smiles. He often becomes irritable, and they are unable to console him. He appears to interact normally with his peers. What is the most likely diagnosis?

A. Posttraumatic stress disorder (PTSD).
B. Autism spectrum disorder.
C. Reactive attachment disorder.
D. Adjustment disorder with depressed mood.
E. Disinhibited social engagement disorder.

9.2 A 6-year-old girl is brought to a child psychiatrist by her new foster parents. She had been removed from her biological parents at an early age because of neglect, and she has been in multiple prior foster homes. Since moving to her new home, her foster parents have noticed that she will initiate conversations with strangers at the supermarket, and she once attempted to go home with another family. During the interview, the child jumps on the psychiatrist's lap and begins stroking her back. Testing has shown that she has a mild intellectual disability, and there is no history of a mood disturbance. What is the best diagnosis?

A. PTSD.
B. Intellectual developmental disorder.

C. Bipolar I disorder.
D. Adjustment disorder with depressed mood.
E. Disinhibited social engagement disorder.

9.3   What is the most common precipitating event for women diagnosed with PTSD?

A. Natural disaster.
B. Experiencing a fire.
C. Sexual assault.
D. Hospitalization in an intensive care unit.
E. Combat.

9.4   Which of the following symptom areas is *not* a required part of the PTSD diagnosis?

A. Reexperiencing of the trauma through intrusive thoughts or dreams.
B. Dissociative symptoms such as derealization or depersonalization.
C. Avoidance of stimuli associated with the event.
D. Negative alterations in mood such as feeling numb or detached from others.
E. Alterations in arousal and reactivity such as irritability/angry outbursts and exaggerated startle response.

9.5   What is the best medication choice for PTSD?

A. Sertraline.
B. Venlafaxine.
C. Diazepam.
D. Prazosin.
E. Lithium.

9.6   A 30-year-old veteran is seen in follow-up for his PTSD precipitated by wartime combat. He reports ongoing disturbing nightmares about his past experiences. He continues to have other symptoms as well, but they are less distressing to him. Which of the following medications is most appropriate to target his chief complaint?

A. Sertraline.
B. Venlafaxine.

C. Clonazepam.

D. Prazosin.

E. Lithium.

9.7   A 24-year-old man seeks help of a psychiatrist because of problems with irritability and feeling "on guard" since a motor vehicle accident 2 weeks earlier. Luckily, he only sustained minor injuries, but his vehicle was destroyed. Since the accident, he has felt out of sorts and has had intrusive memories and nightmares about the event. He has been using public transportation to get to work and now avoids going by the scene of the accident. What is the most likely diagnosis?

A. PTSD.

B. Acute stress disorder.

C. Adjustment disorder with anxious features.

D. Unspecified anxiety disorder.

E. None of the above.

9.8   A 17-year-old boy whose parents divorced 2 months earlier is brought to a therapist by his mother. He has always been a good student, but his grades have dropped, and he has been getting into fights at school over the past month. There is no history of behavioral problems. He says that he isn't depressed, and there have been no changes in his appetite, sleep, or activity level. He answers "I don't know," to most of the therapist's questions. What is the most likely diagnosis?

A. PTSD.

B. Acute stress disorder.

C. Adjustment disorder.

D. Major depression.

E. Reactive attachment disorder.

9.9   What is the most common stressor for adults with an adjustment disorder?

A. Divorce or separation.

B. Marital problems.

C. Work problems.

D. Financial problems.

E. Moving.

9.10 What is the most common stressor to precipitate an adjustment disorder in adolescents?

A. Marital problems in parents.
B. School problems.
C. Drug or alcohol problem.
D. Parental rejection.
E. Boyfriend/girlfriend problems.

9.11 Which of the following is required for a diagnosis of adjustment disorder?

A. Identifiable stressor.
B. Depressive symptoms.
C. Anxious symptoms.
D. Disturbance of conduct.
E. None of the above.

9.12 What is the best treatment for an adjustment disorder?

A. Sedative-hypnotics.
B. SSRIs.
C. Antipsychotics.
D. Supportive therapy.
E. Cognitive-behavioral therapy.

CHAPTER 10

Somatic Symptom Disorders and Dissociative Disorders

10.1 A 30-year-old man presents to his primary care physician with a new concern that he may have a brain tumor. He reports that for the past week he has had tingling on his scalp. He had a mild headache the day before that resolved with ibuprofen. At his last visit a few months ago, he was concerned that he had pancreatic cancer because he noticed a small area of yellow discoloration on his upper arm. What is the most likely diagnosis?

A. Somatic symptom disorder.
B. Illness anxiety disorder.
C. Factitious disorder.
D. Conversion disorder.
E. Malingering.

10.2 A 24-year-old woman is referred to neurology for evaluation of spells that began 2 months earlier. She reports having seizures two or three times a week that are characterized by bilateral arm flap-

Note that most vignettes in this chapter take place in a primary care setting because primary care physicians are more likely to see patients with somatic symptom disorder than are psychiatrists. Patients with these conditions tend not to view them as being psychologically motivated and so rarely seek mental health care for the conditions.

ping without impairment of consciousness or loss of bowel or bladder control. The electroencephalogram is negative for epileptiform activity, and routine laboratory studies are unremarkable. What is the most likely diagnosis?

A. Somatic symptom disorder.
B. Convulsive disorder.
C. Factitious disorder.
D. Conversion disorder.
E. Malingering.

10.3 How many somatic symptoms are required to make a DSM-5 diagnosis of somatic symptom disorder?

A. One.
B. Two.
C. Four.
D. Six.
E. Eight.

10.4 A 60-year-old man on disability sees his family physician in follow-up for chronic pain. He reports pain in multiple joints, and he frequently requests more opioid pain medications to help with his symptoms. Diagnostic studies show only changes consistent with normal aging. The patient's primary concern is with pain, and there is no evidence that he misuses his medications. He has been amenable to trying interventions such as physical therapy, although they have not produced adequate results. What is the most likely diagnosis?

A. Pain disorder.
B. Somatic symptom disorder.
C. Opioid use disorder.
D. Conversion disorder.
E. Malingering.

10.5 A 19-year-old man presents to his family physician, convinced that his intestines are rotting and that he may already be dead. He is not able to cite any symptoms that give rise to this conviction. Physical examination and routine laboratory tests are normal. The patient does not accept his physician's reassurance that he is healthy. What is the most likely diagnosis?

A. Somatic symptom disorder.

B. Illness anxiety disorder.

C. Schizophrenia.

D. Malingering.

E. Unspecified somatic symptom disorder.

10.6   A psychiatrist is asked to consult on a 25-year-old man admitted to a general neurological service for sudden onset of lower-extremity weakness. The patient has reported that he cannot walk, although diagnostic studies have not shown any physical reason to account for the symptoms. The patient asks if he will ever get any better. How should the psychiatrist respond?

A. "Your condition will most likely improve with time."

B. "You will most likely have permanent disability."

C. "Your prognosis is guarded."

D. "It is too early to draw any conclusion."

E. "It will depend on your willingness to engage in cognitive-behavioral therapy."

10.7   A 55-year-old woman sees her family physician for an annual physical examination. During the review of symptoms, she reports chronic dyspepsia. She had the same complaint during her last three visits. She has not had any visits or phone calls between visits. A medical workup for this complaint was negative 3 years ago. She is not preoccupied with this symptom, and her social and occupational functioning is normal. The physician considers diagnosing somatic symptom disorder because there is no obvious medical explanation for her complaint. Her medical student, fresh from her psychiatry clerkship, objects and says that it would inappropriate. Why so?

A. Patients with somatic symptom disorder must have multiple somatic complaints.

B. The patient's lack of interest in her symptoms makes a conversion disorder more likely.

C. The physician has not investigated possible motivations for secondary gain or to play the patient role.

D. The diagnosis of somatic symptom disorder requires the patient have significant preoccupation or personal investment in his or her symptoms.

E. The medical student is wrong, and it is appropriate to diagnose this patient with somatic symptom disorder.

10.8　What is the recommended treatment for somatic symptom disorder?

   A. Selective serotonin reuptake inhibitors (SSRIs).
   B. Benzodiazepine tranquilizers.
   C. Regularly scheduled visits with the same physician.
   D. Referral to specialists in order to provide higher levels of care.
   E. Aggressive workups to offer greater reassurance to patients.

10.9　A psychiatrist is asked to see a 25-year-old man with chronic renal failure admitted to a general medical floor for complications resulting from poor compliance with recommended dialysis. He shows a fair understanding of his medical condition but reports that he just feels like taking a day off from dialysis every now and again. Further interview doesn't reveal clear evidence of depression, anxiety, cognitive impairment, psychosis, or personality disorder. What is the most likely diagnosis?

   A. Psychological factors affecting another medical condition.
   B. Factitious disorder.
   C. Malingering.
   D. Unspecified depressive disorder.
   E. Somatic symptom disorder.

10.10　A psychiatrist is called to see a 25-year-old man with chronic renal failure admitted to a general medical floor for complications resulting from poor compliance with recommended dialysis. He has demanded to leave against medical advice. He has been threatening and verbally abusing staff members. He has fair understanding of his medical condition and is not delirious or confused. Review of his background shows a long history of legal and disciplinary problems dating to childhood. What is the best diagnosis?

   A. Psychological factors affecting another medical condition.
   B. Antisocial personality disorder.
   C. Malingering.
   D. Unspecified depressive disorder.
   E. Somatic symptom disorder.

10.11　A 10-year-old boy receives a couple of new video games for his birthday. The following day he tells his mother that he does not feel up to going to school because of stomach upset, although he appears well. His mother gives him a thermometer to check his temperature and leaves the room. When she comes back, the thermometer shows a temperature of 112 degrees. What is the most likely diagnosis?

A. Factitious disorder.
B. Malingering.
C. Somatic symptom disorder.
D. Separation anxiety disorder.
E. Psychological factors affecting another medical condition.

10.12 Which personality disorder is frequently comorbid with dissociative identity disorder?

A. Schizotypal personality disorder.
B. Schizoid personality disorder.
C. Dependent personality disorder.
D. Borderline personality disorder.
E. Narcissistic personality disorder.

10.13 What is the standard treatment for depersonalization/derealization disorder?

A. Benzodiazepine tranquilizers.
B. Fluoxetine.
C. Second-generation antipsychotic.
D. Psychotherapy.
E. There is no standard treatment for depersonalization/derealization disorder.

10.14 A 19-year-old college student reports that for the past 2 weeks, since smoking cannabis for the first time, she has felt cut off from herself. She says that she feels she is watching herself go through the motions, and feels unable to connect with her experiences. She did not feel this way prior to smoking cannabis. What is the best diagnosis?

A. Dissociative identity disorder.
B. Depersonalization/derealization disorder.
C. Dissociative amnesia.
D. Substance-induced mood disorder.
E. Schizophrenia.

10.15 A 35-year-old man presents to the emergency room. He shows the staff his driver's license and requests help because he has forgotten who he is and where he lives. His driver's license shows that he lives in a town over 100 miles away. A medical workup including brain imaging is unremarkable. Neuropsychological assessment shows gaps in his ability to recall autobiographical information, but formal testing of memory is normal. What is the most likely diagnosis?

A. Dissociative identity disorder.
B. Depersonalization/derealization disorder.
C. Dissociative amnesia.
D. Posttraumatic stress disorder.
E. Factitious disorder.

— CHAPTER 11 —

Feeding and Eating Disorders

11.1 A mother reports to a pediatrician that her 4-year-old son has been eating small quantities of dirt and pebbles from the garden at home. What is the most likely diagnosis?

A. Pica.
B. Rumination disorder.
C. Avoidant/restrictive food intake disorder.
D. Other specified feeding disorder.
E. None of the above.

11.2 A mother reports to a pediatrician that her 15-month-old daughter mouths on a variety of inanimate objects in the home. What is the most likely diagnosis?

A. Pica.
B. Rumination disorder.
C. Avoidant/restrictive food intake disorder.
D. Other specified feeding disorder.
E. None of the above.

11.3 A 7-year-old child is brought to a pediatric gastroenterologist by her parents. They are concerned because they have noticed that the child has been regurgitating swallowed food, and then swallowing it again or sometimes expelling it. The child does not report symptoms such as heartburn or stomach pain. Her food intake is appropriate for her age, and she does not appear preoccupied with her body shape or size. A medical workup is unremarkable. What is the most likely diagnosis?

A. Pica.
B. Rumination disorder.
C. Avoidant/restrictive food intake disorder.
D. Bulimia nervosa.
E. Anorexia nervosa.

11.4   An 11-year-old boy with autism spectrum disorder is brought to a pediatrician because his mother is concerned about his poor appetite. He has always been a picky eater, but his mother is especially concerned because it's about time for his "growth spurt." The boy is thin but not emaciated and is of normal height. He tells his doctor that he's not very interested in food and that he finds the textures of most foods unappetizing. He denies preoccupation with being thin, and there is no evidence of depression. What is the most likely diagnosis?

A. Pica.
B. Rumination disorder.
C. Avoidant/restrictive food intake disorder.
D. Bulimia nervosa.
E. Anorexia nervosa.

11.5   A 50-year-old man is brought to his family physician at his wife's insistence. She is concerned because he has lost 15 lbs. in the past month. He "barely eats a thing," she says. The man reports he no longer has any interest in anything. He spends most of the day watching TV but doesn't pay much attention to the programs. He complains of poor sleep, waking up at about 3 A.M. every morning and not being able to go back to sleep. He displays a restricted affect. What is the most likely diagnosis?

A. Pica.
B. Rumination disorder.
C. Avoidant/restrictive food intake disorder.
D. Major depressive disorder.
E. Anorexia nervosa.

11.6 What is the key difference between anorexia nervosa and bulimia nervosa?

A. Presence of binging behavior.
B. Presence of purging behavior.
C. Preoccupation with one's body weight.
D. Current body weight.
E. Personality of the patient.

11.7 Which of the following physical examination findings is *not* typical of anorexia nervosa?

A. Tachycardia.
B. Hypokalemia.
C. Amenorrhea.
D. Hair loss.
E. Constipation.

11.8 Which brain region plays an important role in regulating feeding behavior?

A. Thalamus.
B. Hypothalamus.
C. Pineal gland.
D. Amygdala.
E. Entorhinal cortex.

11.9 Which of the following physical examination findings would suggest a diagnosis of bulimia nervosa or the binge-purge subtype of anorexia nervosa rather than another eating disorder?

A. Constipation.
B. Decreased thyroid-stimulating hormone.
C. Calluses on the dorsal surface of the hands.
D. Amenorrhea.
E. Hair loss.

11.10 During a routine health maintenance exam, a 30-year-old man tells his family physician that he has been having trouble losing weight. He reports that 3–4 times each week, he loses control of his eating and consumes a very large quantity of food such that he feels physically uncomfortable afterward. He feels embarrassed, and because of this tendency he makes up excuses to reject dinner invitations. He is overweight and has some concern about his body image, but he denies being obsessed with being thin. He denies excessive exercise or other compensatory behaviors. What is the most likely diagnosis?

A. Binge-eating disorder.
B. Rumination disorder.
C. Avoidant/restrictive food intake disorder.
D. Bulimia nervosa.
E. Anorexia nervosa.

11.11 Which antidepressant is contraindicated in patients with eating disorders?

A. Fluoxetine.
B. Sertraline.
C. Bupropion.
D. Venlafaxine.
E. Mirtazapine.

11.12 Which medication is U.S. Food and Drug Administration (FDA) approved for the treatment of bulimia nervosa?

A. Sertraline.
B. Fluoxetine.
C. Lithium.
D. Venlafaxine.
E. Olanzapine.

11.13 What is the first objective in treating a patient with an eating disorder?

A. Correct faulty cognitions about body image.
B. Modify distorted eating behaviors.
C. Restore nutritional status.
D. Correct unhealthy home environment that gives rise to the disorder.
E. Initiate SSRI to address disrupted serotonergic neurotransmission.

⊢CHAPTER 12⊣

Sleep-Wake Disorders

12.1 Which sleep stage is characterized by rapid conjugate eye movements, penile/clitoral engorgement, and reduced muscle tone?

A. Stage 0.
B. Stage 1.
C. Stage 2.
D. Stage 3.
E. Rapid eye movement (REM) sleep.

12.2 Which procedure can be used to measure excessive sleepiness?

A. Polysomnography.
B. Multiple Sleep Latency Test.
C. Electroencephalogram (EEG).
D. Clinical sleep hygiene assessment.
E. Neuropsychological evaluation.

12.3 Which of the following is *not* a routine sleep hygiene recommendation?

A. Discontinuing the intake of alcohol, caffeine, and sedative-hypnotics.
B. Avoiding reading, working, or watching TV in bed.
C. Staying awake in bed for long periods of time until sleep onset occurs.
D. Going to bed and waking up at the same time every day, even on weekends.
E. Avoiding napping.

12.4　Which of the following can be used to treat insomnia disorder?

    A. Temazepam.
    B. Trazodone.
    C. Diphenhydramine.
    D. Zolpidem.
    E. All of the above.

12.5　A 35-year-old man complains to his family physician of difficulty falling asleep for the past 8 months. It takes him up to an hour to fall asleep, and he reports feeling fatigued throughout the day. He sometimes feels irritable but denies significant depression. He does not snore, nor does he feel sleepy during the day. He stopped his caffeine intake a couple of months ago after reading about sleep hygiene on the Internet. What is the most likely diagnosis?

    A. Hypersomnolence disorder.
    B. Narcolepsy.
    C. Insomnia disorder.
    D. Obstructive sleep apnea.
    E. Other specified insomnia disorder.

12.6　Which of the following suggests hypersomnolence disorder rather than narcolepsy?

    A. Daytime napping.
    B. Decreased REM sleep latency.
    C. Spells of brief loss of muscle tone (hypotonia).
    D. Hypocretin deficiency.
    E. Sleep inertia.

12.7　A 22-year-old woman presents to a sleep disorders clinic. She reports that she is groggy most every morning and it takes her over an hour to become alert. She sleeps 9–10 hours at night. She feels sleepy during the day and will sometimes take a 1- to 2-hour nap. She denies episodes of cataplexy or excessive caffeine use. Which treatment may be effective for this patient?

    A. Selective serotonin reuptake inhibitor.
    B. Benzodiazepine.
    C. Stimulant.

D. Nonbenzodiazepine hypnotic.

E. Antihistamine.

12.8 What causes narcolepsy?

A. Loss of cholinergic cells in the nucleus basalis.

B. Loss of hypocretin-secreting cells in the hypothalamus.

C. Decrease in REM latency.

D. Poor sleep hygiene.

E. The cause is unknown.

12.9 Which of the following is an effective treatment for sleep attacks associated with narcolepsy?

A. Tricyclic antidepressant.

B. Sodium oxybate.

C. Methylphenidate.

D. Zolpidem.

E. Improved sleep hygiene.

12.10 What is the technical term used for a decrease in airflow during sleeping?

A. Apnea.

B. Hypopnea.

C. Hyperpnea.

D. Tachypnea.

E. Hyperpnoea.

12.11 A 45-year-old obese man complains to his family physician of chronic trouble with sleep maintenance. He falls asleep easily at night, but awakens 10–20 times throughout the night. He feels fatigued during the day and occasionally takes short naps. He says his wife tells him that he snores loudly at times but not on most nights. He sleeps in a quiet dark room and goes to bed at about the same time on most nights, but on the weekend he might stay up 30–45 minutes later than usual. His blood pressure is normal. He drinks 2–3 cups of coffee in the morning and may have a 12 oz. can of soda in the late afternoon. What is the best next step in management of this patient?

A. Prescribe a benzodiazepine.
B. Have the patient eliminate caffeine intake.
C. Administer Multiple Sleep Latency Test.
D. Administer polysomnogram.
E. Counsel the patient on sleep hygiene and follow-up in 3 months.

12.12 Which of the following is *not* suggestive of obstructive sleep apnea?

A. Snoring.
B. Daytime fatigue.
C. Apneic episodes.
D. Crescendo-decrescendo variation in tidal volume.
E. Difficulty to controlling hypertension.

12.13 Which of the following treatment methods can be used for refractory cases of obstructive sleep apnea?

A. Weight-loss counseling.
B. Continuous positive airway pressure (CPAP).
C. Sedative-hypnotics.
D. Acetazolamide.
E. Uvulopalatopharyngoplasty.

12.14 Which medication can be used to stimulate breathing in patients with central sleep apnea?

A. Sodium oxybate.
B. Chloral hydrate.
C. Acetazolamide.
D. Zolpidem.
E. Any benzodiazepine.

12.15 A 50-year-old woman with chronic obstructive pulmonary disease reports to her family physician that she has morning headache and daytime fatigue. Routine laboratory studies are remarkable for elevated CO_2. Polysomnogram shows periods of decreased respiration. What is the most likely diagnosis?

A. Obstructive sleep apnea.
B. Central sleep apnea.
C. Sleep-related hypoventilation.

D. Hypersomnolence disorder.

E. Narcolepsy.

12.16 A 27-year-old man who works nights at a convenience store reports to his family physician that his energy is chronically low and he has little motivation. He can only sleep 4–6 hours during the day. He tries to maintain a diurnal schedule on his days off on the weekend but has trouble falling asleep at night. What is the most likely diagnosis?

A. Insomnia disorder.

B. Obstructive sleep apnea.

C. Hypersomnolence disorder.

D. Circadian rhythm sleep-wake disorder.

E. Narcolepsy.

12.17 What is the best treatment for circadian rhythm sleep-wake disorder, shift work type?

A. Improved sleep hygiene.

B. Methylphenidate to improve alertness.

C. Zolpidem to assist with daytime sleep.

D. Melatonin to regulate circadian rhythm.

E. Discontinue shift work.

12.18 What is the DSM-5 diagnosis used for both sleep walking and sleep terrors?

A. Non-REM (NREM) sleep arousal disorder.

B. REM sleep behavior disorder.

C. Parasomnia.

D. Circadian rhythm sleep-wake disorder.

E. None of the above.

12.19 A 15-year-old boy has recurrent vivid dreams with frightening violent content. He wakes up in the morning with a racing heart and heavy breathing, but he does not scream or act out. What is the most likely diagnosis?

A. REM sleep behavior disorder.

B. NREM sleep arousal disorder, sleep terror type.

C. Nightmare disorder.

D. Parasomnia.

E. None of the above.

12.20 Which sleep disorder is associated with Parkinson's disease, Lewy body dementia, and multiple systems atrophy?

A. REM sleep behavior disorder.

B. NREM sleep arousal disorder, sleep terror type.

C. Nightmare disorder.

D. Parasomnia.

E. Central sleep apnea.

12.21 A 31-year-old woman reports to her family physician that she has the uncomfortable sensation of having to move her legs at night when she is in bed. She says she does not sleep well because of this. She wonders if something can be given to treat her condition. Which of the following can be used to treat this condition?

A. Zolpidem.

B. Pramipexole.

C. L-Dopa.

D. Clonazepam.

E. Imipramine.

⊢ CHAPTER 13 ⊣

Sexual Dysfunction, Gender Dysphoria, and Paraphilias

13.1 How long should a disorder of sexual function be present prior to diagnosis?

    A. At least 18 months.
    B. At least 4 months.
    C. At least 1 month.
    D. At least 6 months.
    E. At least 1 year.

13.2 Which of the following would preclude a diagnosis of a sexual dysfunction?

    A. Severe relationship stress.
    B. A nonsexual mental disorder that would account for symptoms.
    C. Disturbance caused by substance use or medication.
    D. Disturbance caused by medical condition such as diabetes.
    E. Any of the above would preclude diagnosis.

13.3 A 22-year-old man reports to his family physician that he has had persistent difficulty achieving orgasm during intercourse with his partner. He has no trouble attaining an erection. The problem has been ongoing since the relationship began about a year ago. He does not have any difficulty achieving orgasm during masturbation and reports that otherwise his relationship is going well. He does not take any medications. What is the most likely diagnosis?

A. No diagnosis.
B. Other specified sexual dysfunction.
C. Delayed ejaculation.
D. Male hypoactive sexual desire disorder.
E. Erectile disorder.

13.4 A 28-year-old man reports to his family physician that he has had persistent difficulty achieving orgasm both with his partner and while masturbating. He has no trouble attaining an erection. His problem has been ongoing since the relationship began about a year ago. He reports that otherwise his relationship is going well. He does not take any medications except for fluoxetine. What is the most likely diagnosis?

A. Medication-induced sexual dysfunction.
B. Other specified sexual dysfunction.
C. Delayed ejaculation.
D. Male hypoactive sexual desire disorder.
E. Erectile disorder.

13.5 A 40-year-old man with type 2 diabetes mellitus reports to his family physician that he has progressive difficulty achieving an erection prior to intercourse with his wife. He continues to experience spontaneous erections at times when he is not planning to have intercourse. What is the most likely etiology of the patient's problem?

A. Secondary to type 2 diabetes mellitus.
B. Secondary to psychological factors.
C. Secondary to marital discord.
D. Secondary to a medical condition other than type 2 diabetes.
E. Unable to determine without more information.

13.6 A 30-year-old woman reports to her family physician of ongoing sexual difficulties with her partner for the last several years. She experiences vaginal and pelvic pain during intercourse. She denies that there is difficulty achieving vaginal penetration, and she is not sure about tightening of her pelvic muscles during penetration. What is the most likely diagnosis?

A. Dyspareunia.
B. Vaginismus.
C. Genito-pelvic pain disorder.
D. Female sexual interest/arousal disorder.
E. None of the above.

13.7 A 50-year-old man reports to his family physician that in the past few months he has had a new onset of premature ejaculation during intercourse. He is baffled about why it is happening at his age. He has been feeling more jittery than usual over the past few months, and he reports occasional palpitations and diaphoresis on review of systems. What is the next best step in management of this patient?

A. Refer to a psychiatrist.
B. Start a selective serotonin reuptake inhibitor (SSRI).
C. Refer to a psychotherapist.
D. Order thyroid-stimulating hormone.
E. None of the above.

13.8 What medication can be used to treat premature ejaculation?

A. Sildenafil.
B. Alprostadil.
C. Vardenafil.
D. Paroxetine.
E. Tadalafil.

13.9 Which of the following medications is a standard treatment for erectile disorder?

A. Vardenafil.
B. Paroxetine.
C. Dibucaine.
D. Testosterone.
E. Topical estrogen.

13.10 Which of the following is *not* typical of gender dysphoria?

A. Onset occurs in childhood.
B. The child prefers to play with children of the same gender.
C. The child expresses a strong desire to be rid of one's primary

and secondary sexual characteristics because of incongruence between one's expressed and experienced gender.

D. The child expresses strong preference for cross-sex roles in make-believe play.

E. The child shows a strong preference for games, toys, and activities stereotypically associated with the opposite gender.

13.11 A 40-year-old man reports to his psychiatrist that he enjoys dressing in women's clothing prior to intercourse, but this has caused conflict with his wife. He identifies himself as heterosexual, and he reports he is comfortable being male. What is the best diagnosis?

A. Gender dysphoria.
B. Transvestic disorder.
C. Voyeuristic disorder.
D. Exhibitionistic disorder.
E. Frotteuristic disorder.

13.12 What is the DSM-5 term for an anomalous sexual activity preference?

A. Paraphilic disorder.
B. Paraphilia.
C. Infantilism.
D. Infantilism disorder.
E. None of the above.

13.13 What is the standard treatment for paraphilic disorders?

A. SSRI.
B. Leuprolide.
C. Naltrexone.
D. Cognitive-behavioral therapy.
E. Medroxyprogesterone.

CHAPTER 14

Disruptive, Impulse-Control, and Conduct Disorders

14.1 A 7-year-old girl is brought to a therapist by her mother. Her mother says that the girl is always touchy and irritable and gets very angry when she is told to do anything. The behavior has been present for over a year. When asked about her symptoms, the girl says that it's her mother's fault for always making her mad. She has not engaged in any stealing, fire setting, or runaway behavior. She gets along with her peers, and her grades in school are good. What is the most likely diagnosis?

A. Antisocial personality disorder.
B. Conduct disorder.
C. Attention deficit/hyperactivity disorder.
D. Oppositional defiant disorder.
E. Normal development.

14.2 A 16-year-old boy with an autism spectrum disorder is brought to the emergency room by his family. His father reports that he broke two windows and smashed several plates in the kitchen after his father told him that he would not be able to use the computer for the next day because he had failed to clean up his room. The boy has had similar destructive outbursts when his computer privileges have been restricted in the past. Ordinarily, he is quiet, keeps to himself, and does not bother others. He does not have a history of truancy, fire setting, cruelty to animals, or fighting. What is the most likely diagnosis?

A. Oppositional defiant disorder.

B. Conduct disorder.

C. Antisocial personality disorder.

D. Intermittent explosive disorder.

E. No additional diagnosis apart from autism spectrum disorder.

14.3 A 16-year-old boy is brought to a psychiatrist at his parents' insistence for problem behavior ongoing for 3 years. He has had repeated legal trouble for acts of vandalism, and he has been expelled from school several times for fighting. He is failing all of his classes. He tells the psychiatrist that he doesn't care about his school work and has no remorse for his actions. What DSM-5 specifier is appropriate for this form of conduct disorder?

A. With limited prosocial emotions.

B. With antisocial personality features.

C. With psychopathic personality features.

D. Childhood-onset type.

E. DSM-5 does not have a descriptor for such cases.

14.4 A 35-year-old man is charged with arson after burning down a building he owned in order to collect insurance money. He has no previous criminal history, and his work history has been stable. He denies any previous episodes of fire setting. What is the most likely psychiatric diagnosis?

A. Antisocial personality disorder.

B. Adult antisocial behavior.

C. Pyromania.

D. Intermittent explosive disorder.

E. Conduct disorder.

14.5 What is the treatment for pyromania?

A. Cognitive-behavioral therapy.

B. Selective serotonin reuptake inhibitor (SSRI).

C. Mood stabilizer such as carbamazepine.

D. Atypical antipsychotic such as risperidone.

E. There is no standard treatment for pyromania.

14.6 A 24-year-old woman comes forward to establish care with a therapist. She reports a problem with compulsive stealing. She has taken small items of modest value from stores and from the homes of friends and family on many occasions since adolescence. She reports feeling tension before the theft and a sense of gratification afterward. She is motivated to change her behavior because she was recently given probation as a consequence of shoplifting. She denies any other criminal activity or interpersonal problems. What is the most likely diagnosis?

A. Conduct disorder.
B. Antisocial personality disorder.
C. Kleptomania.
D. Adult antisocial behavior.
E. Oppositional defiant disorder.

14.7 All but which of the following may be beneficial for patients with intermittent explosive disorder?

A. Fluoxetine.
B. Oxcarbazepine.
C. Cognitive-behavior therapy.
D. Benzodiazepine tranquilizers.
E. Fluoxetine and oxcarbazepine.

14.8 Naltrexone has shown to be more effective than placebo for treating which of the following?

A. Intermittent explosive disorder.
B. Conduct disorder.
C. Kleptomania.
D. Pyromania.
E. Oppositional defiant disorder.

─CHAPTER 15─

Substance-Related and Addictive Disorders

15.1 A 48-year-old woman reports to her family physician that she has been drinking a bottle of wine two to three times per week for the past 3 years. She has not been successful in her attempts to cut back her drinking, and her drinking has led to conflicts with her family. She has not had any problems at work as the result of her drinking, and she has never had symptoms of alcohol withdrawal. What is the best diagnosis?

A. Alcohol use disorder.
B. Alcohol dependence.
C. Alcohol abuse.
D. Alcoholism.
E. Alcohol abuse disorder.

15.2 How long can cannabis be detected by urine drug screen after last use?

A. 24 hours.
B. 3 days.
C. 1 week.
D. 3 weeks.
E. 6 weeks.

15.3 Which neurotransmitter plays a key role in the development of all substance use disorders?

A. Serotonin.
B. Acetylcholine.

C. β-Endorphin.
D. Norepinephrine.
E. Dopamine.

15.4 Which neurotransmitter plays a role specifically in the development of opioid use disorders?

A. Dopamine.
B. β-Endorphin.
C. Acetylcholine.
D. Serotonin.
E. Norepinephrine.

15.5 A 17-year-old girl is referred for treatment of substance misuse. She smokes cannabis nearly every day and has started to use cocaine a few times a week in the past 2 months. Her father drinks excessively, and the family receives government assistance. One reason she gives for using illegal drugs is that her friends use these substances, and it is hard for her not to go along with them. Which of the following factors associated with this patient is *not* associated with risk of developing a substance use disorder?

A. Low socioeconomic status.
B. Susceptibility to peer influence.
C. Female sex.
D. Age.
E. Parental alcoholism.

15.6 How many positive responses on a CAGE test are needed to indicate that a person may have an alcohol use disorder?

A. One.
B. Two.
C. Three.
D. Four.
E. The CAGE test is not a good screening test for alcohol use disorders.

15.7 Which of the following develops as a late-stage consequence of an alcohol use disorder?

A. Decreased work productivity.
B. Moodiness or irritability.

C. Palmar erythema.

D. Rosacea.

E. Jaundice.

15.8 A 45-year-old man reports a 10-year history of heavy alcohol consumption to his family physician. He tells his physician that he is not as "sharp" as he used to be before he started drinking and that he has some mild difficulties with everyday memory tasks. He asks his doctor if these memory problems will be permanent. What is the best response?

A. "Even if you stop drinking, these memory problems are likely to be irreversible but not progressive."

B. "Even if you stop drinking, these memory problems are likely to be irreversible and progressive."

C. "If you stop drinking now, these memory problems may partially reverse."

D. "If you stop drinking now, your memory will likely fully completely."

E. None of the above.

15.9 What percentage of motor vehicle deaths are related to alcohol?

A. 10%.

B. 20%.

C. 30%.

D. 40%.

E. >50%.

15.10 Which of the following are the last symptoms to develop during the course of severe alcohol withdrawal?

A. Delirium, fever, autonomic hyperarousal.

B. Auditory, visual, tactile hallucinations in the presence of a clear sensorium.

C. Seizures.

D. Anxiety, tremor, nausea.

E. Increased heart rate and blood pressure.

15.11 A psychiatrist is called to evaluate a 38-year-old man for admission to a psychiatric unit for alcohol detoxification and treatment of depression. He has been drinking large quantities of vodka daily for several months. He previously drank 3–4 beers nearly daily for almost 5 years. His last drink was 6 hours ago. He is currently pleasant and cooperative. His is fully oriented and in no distress. The psychiatrist asks the man if he has ever had the delirium tremens. He responds, "Oh yeah, I've got the shakes right now," and he holds out his hands to show the psychiatrist his mild tremor. How shall the psychiatrist proceed?

A. Recommend admission to intensive care because delirium tremens (DTs) can be fatal.
B. Admit the patient to psychiatry for alcohol rehabilitation.
C. Administer chlordiazepoxide now.
D. Collect additional information such as if the man has ever had confusion and fever during withdrawal or had become agitated.
E. None of the above.

15.12 Which medication used to treat alcohol dependence works by inhibiting alcohol dehydrogenase?

A. Naltrexone.
B. Disulfiram.
C. Acamprosate.
D. Chlordiazepoxide.
E. Lorazepam.

15.13 A 20-year-old student sees his internist for anxiety symptoms. He reports that he has started worrying about everything since he started college about 2 years ago. He has trouble falling asleep and staying asleep nearly every night. His mood is mildly irritable, and he appears restless. He does not smoke, use alcohol, or use illicit drugs. He reports that he drinks eight or more cups of coffee daily to help him stay motivated when studying, with his last cup around 8–10 P.M. What is the most likely diagnosis?

A. Generalized anxiety disorder.
B. Bipolar I disorder.
C. Caffeine-induced anxiety disorder.
D. Panic disorder.
E. Insomnia disorder.

15.14 Which of the following is *not* associated with cannabis use?

    A. Increased risk of developing schizophrenia.
    B. Increased risk of smoking cigarettes and abusing other drugs.
    C. Tachycardia, dry mouth, and conjunctivitis during intoxication.
    D. Flashbacks between periods of use.
    E. Feeling that time has slowed and increased appetite during intoxication.

15.15 A 19-year-old man presents to the emergency room complaining of acute-onset severe anxiety, confusion, time expansion, and vivid visual hallucinations. He took LSD for the first time 3 hours ago and is very uncomfortable, but he is cooperative in interview. His pupils are dilated, and he has mild tachycardia. Reassurance does not succeed in calming him down. What is the next best step in managing this case?

    A. Give an antipsychotic.
    B. Give a benzodiazepine.
    C. Give clonidine.
    D. Give naltrexone.
    E. Refer the man to a substance use treatment program.

15.16 A 30-year-old man requests help for an opioid abuse disorder. He has used large quantities of prescription narcotics obtained on the streets and will also inject heroin when it is available. He has tried to quit these drugs on his own several times without success. Which of the following is the best option to treat his opioid use disorder and reduce his risk of relapse and criminal activity?

    A. Referral to Narcotics Anonymous.
    B. Detoxification with clonidine followed by outpatient counseling.
    C. Referral to a methadone maintenance program.
    D. Prescribing naltrexone.
    E. Detoxification with clonidine followed by referral to an intensive outpatient program.

15.17 A 26-year-old woman comes to your office seeking help for anxiety and panic attacks. She was last seen by your colleague a week ago, but she reports that she has lost her prescription for alprazolam. She asks you to write a new prescription for alprazolam 3 mg four times daily. She reports that nothing else works and that she has allergies to the selective serotonin reuptake inhibitors. Which of the following is *not* a valid reason to have serious concerns about prescribing alprazolam to this patient?

A. Concern about doctor-shopping behavior.
B. Report that "nothing else works."
C. Report of severe allergies to other medications commonly used to treat anxiety.
D. Report of a lost prescription.
E. Lethality of benzodiazepines in overdose.

15.18 A 23-year-old man with no previous psychiatric history is brought to the emergency room by the police for agitated and disorganized behavior. He is paranoid and believes that the government is sending him messages through a microchip that was implanted in one of his teeth. He has not slept for 3 days. He is distractible in interview but otherwise oriented. A urine drug screen is positive for amphetamine. He is otherwise medically stable and is admitted to the psychiatry unit. What is the best course of treatment for this patient's psychotic symptoms?

A. Supportive care and possibly short-term use of antipsychotic.
B. Antipsychotic therapy for 6 months.
C. Cognitive-behavioral psychotherapy.
D. Imipramine.
E. Lithium.

15.19 What form of therapy for substance use disorders rewards patients for appropriate behavior (e.g., giving patients who submit clean urine samples vouchers that can be exchanged for retail goods and services)?

A. Contingency management.
B. Motivational interviewing.
C. Cognitive-behavioral therapy.
D. Behavioral activation.
E. Twelve-step program.

15.20 Which of the following treatments has a role in treating gambling disorder?

A. Gamblers Anonymous (GA).
B. Naltrexone.
C. Motivational interviewing.
D. Cognitive-behavioral therapy (CBT).
E. All of the above.

CHAPTER 16

Neurocognitive Disorders

16.1 Which of the following is a diagnostic category (or categories) new to DSM-5 for the diagnosis of neurocognitive disorders?

A. Social cognitive disorder.
B. Major neurocognitive disorder.
C. Major cognitive impairment disorder.
D. Mild neurocognitive disorder.
E. Major neurocognitive and mild neurocognitive disorders.

16.2 Processing speed is a part of which cognitive domain?

A. Social cognition.
B. Complex attention.
C. Learning and memory.
D. Executive function.
E. Language.

16.3 Which of the following is *not* a risk factor for delirium?

A. Use of narcotics.
B. Recent surgery.
C. Older age.
D. Preexisting depression.
E. Systemic infection.

16.4 Which of the following is *least* consistent with delirium?

A. Fluctuation in mental status throughout the day.
B. Disturbance of memory.

C. Occurrence in a hospitalized patient receiving high doses of narcotics.

D. Patient reports of visual and tactile hallucinations.

E. Insidious onset.

16.5 In which of the following patients with delirium is a benzodiazepine *least* likely to worsen delirium?

A. A highly agitated 25-year-old man hospitalized for 2 weeks for encephalopathy.

B. A calm 32-year-old woman hospitalized for 1 week for pneumonia.

C. A 65-year-old alcoholic man hospitalized for the past 3 days recovering from abdominal surgery.

D. An agitated 75-year-old woman with sepsis who reports vivid visual hallucinations.

E. Any patient with delirium.

16.6 Which of the following would distinguish a major neurocognitive disorder from a mild neurocognitive disorder?

A. Decline in memory from baseline.

B. Presence of word finding difficulties.

C. Presence of impairment on neuropsychological assessment.

D. Acute onset over days.

E. Impairment in ability to live independently.

16.7 What percentage of patients with Alzheimer's disease develop psychotic symptoms such as hallucinations and delusions as their illness progresses?

A. 1%.

B. 5%.

C. 10%.

D. 25%.

E. 50%.

16.8 A 67-year-old retired accountant presents to his family physician accompanied by his wife. His wife reports that he has been having progressive difficulty remembering appointments and important dates over the past 2 years, and she no longer allows him to drive. There are no current safety concerns at home. Brief cog-

nitive assessment shows that he has impairment in short-term recall and has difficulty drawing a clock. What is the next best step
in management of this case?

A. Referral to a skilled nursing facility.
B. Medical workup.
C. Neuropsychological assessment.
D. Start donepezil.
E. Referral to a psychiatrist to confirm diagnosis of neurocogni-
tive disorder.

16.9 Which test can distinguish Alzheimer's disease from other neurocognitive disorders?

A. Magnetic resonance imaging (MRI).
B. Functional MRI.
C. Fluorodeoxyglucose positron emission tomography (PET)
scan.
D. Lumbar puncture.
E. Alzheimer's disease can only be confirmed on autopsy.

16.10 A 59-year-old woman is brought to her family physician accompanied by her spouse. She has had worsening of short-term memory and progressive apathy over the past month. She also reports
low mood, insomnia, and low appetite, and she has lost 10 lbs.
since the symptoms begin. She answers "I don't know" to many
basic questions on a brief cognitive assessment. Which of the following medications would be of most benefit to this patient?

A. Donepezil.
B. Tacrine.
C. Sertraline.
D. Aripiprazole.
E. Memantine.

16.11 Which of the following is most specific for Alzheimer's disease?

A. Neurofibrillary tangles.
B. β-Amyloid plaques.
C. Hyperphosphorylated tau protein.
D. Apolipoprotein E polymorphism.
E. All of the above are equally specific changes.

16.12 Primary progressive aphasia and a behavioral-variant subtype occur in which neurocognitive disorder?

A. Alzheimer's disease.
B. Frontotemporal neurocognitive disorder.
C. Neurocognitive disorder with Lewy bodies.
D. Vascular neurocognitive disorder.
E. None of the above.

16.13 Which neurocognitive disorder is sometimes associated with rapid
eye movement (REM) sleep behavior disorder?

A. Alzheimer's disease.
B. Frontotemporal neurocognitive disorder.
C. Neurocognitive disorder with Lewy bodies.
D. Vascular neurocognitive disorder.
E. None of the above.

16.14 A 67-year-old man is brought in to see his family physician by his
family. They are concerned because he has had progressive difficulty keeping up with daily chores at home and is more irritable
than usual. He tells the physician that he wouldn't be so irritable
if his wife hadn't moved so many of her friends into the house.
His wife reports that they live alone, and he seems to see people
that aren't there. The patient is oriented and attends to the interview without difficulty. The physician notices that the patient has
a shuffling gait. What is the most likely diagnosis?

A. Alzheimer's disease.
B. Frontotemporal neurocognitive disorder.
C. Neurocognitive disorder with Lewy bodies.
D. Vascular neurocognitive disorder.
E. Dementia.

16.15 A rapid, progressive stepwise cognitive decline suggests which
neurocognitive disorder?

A. Alzheimer's disease.
B. Frontotemporal neurocognitive disorder.
C. Neurocognitive disorder with Lewy bodies.
D. Vascular neurocognitive disorder.
E. Delirium.

16.16 A 25-year-old man recently diagnosed with an HIV infection sees his internist to address some concerns. He has read about "HIV dementia," and he asks his physician about his risk of developing this complication. What is the most accurate response?

A. It's a rare complication, so your risk is low.
B. You have a high risk of developing this condition at some point.
C. We can't determine this at the present.
D. There's a fair chance you may eventually develop some mild cognitive problems, but your risk of developing severe cognitive problems is low.
E. None of the above.

16.17 Which of the following findings is characteristic of Creutzfeldt-Jakob disease?

A. Triphasic complexes on electroencephalogram (EEG).
B. Diffuse slowing on EEG.
C. Hypocretin deficiency.
D. Degeneration of the mammillary bodies.
E. Hypometabolism of parietal and temporal areas on PET scan.

16.18 Dementia, gait disturbance, and urinary incontinence are the classic triad of which medical condition that can cause a neurocognitive disorder?

A. Pellagra.
B. Prion disease.
C. Subdural hematoma.
D. Alcohol use.
E. Normal pressure hydrocephalus.

16.19 Which of the following medications is an appropriate choice to help with nighttime agitation, or "sundowning," in patients with neurocognitive disorders?

A. Lithium.
B. Carbamazepine.
C. Divalproex.
D. Trazodone.
E. Chlorpromazine.

16.20 Which of the following cognitive-enhancing drugs works on *N*-methyl-D-aspartate (NMDA) receptors?

A. Donepezil.
B. Tacrine.
C. Memantine.
D. Rivastigmine.
E. Galantamine.

16.21 Why has the U.S. Food and Drug Administration (FDA) issued a black box warning about the use of second-generation antipsychotics in elderly patients with neurocognitive disorders?

A. They are associated with an increased rate of cognitive decline.
B. They are associated with severe gastrointestinal side effects.
C. They are associated with an increased risk of mortality.
D. Liver enzymes must be monitored regularly.
E. They have no benefit for managing disruptive behaviors in patients with neurocognitive disorders.

CHAPTER 17

Personality Disorders

17.1 Which was the first DSM to include disturbances of personality?

  A. DSM-I.
  B. DSM-II.
  C. DSM-III.
  D. DSM-IV.
  E. DSM-5.

17.2 Which of the following is *not* true of the general criteria of a personality disorder?

  A. The behavior is consistent with the individual's cultural expectations.
  B. It is stable over time, with onset in adolescence or early adulthood.
  C. The disorder leads to distress or impairment.
  D. The disorder is not limited to episodes of illness.
  E. All of the above are part of the general criteria of a personality disorder.

17.3 A patient has long-standing discrete episodes of mania and depression dating to late adolescence. During manic episodes, he displays elevated mood, decreased sleep, pressured speech, and flight of ideas. The episodes typically result in psychiatric hospitalization. During the manic episodes, he engages in antisocial behavior, including committing assaults and writing bad checks. He is a quiet, law-abiding citizen between episodes of mania. What is the best diagnosis?

A. Antisocial personality disorder.
B. Bipolar I disorder.
C. Personality disorder due to bipolar disorder.
D. Bipolar I disorder plus antisocial personality disorder.
E. None of the above.

17.4 A patient has long-standing discrete episodes of mania and depression dating back to late adolescence. During the manic episodes, he has elevated mood, decreased sleep, pressured speech, and flight of ideas that typically result in psychiatric hospitalization. He gets into more legal trouble than usual during these periods, but even during periods of euthymia, he tends to engage in illegal activities such as shoplifting and burglary. He has done so since early adolescence, and he does not show any remorse for these actions. How would you best diagnose this patient?

A. Antisocial personality disorder.
B. Bipolar I disorder.
C. Personality disorder due to bipolar disorder.
D. Bipolar affective disorder type 1 plus antisocial personality disorder.
E. None of the above.

17.5 Which of the following does *not* represent a major personality trait according to personality theorists who favor a dimensional perspective?

A. Extraversion.
B. Agreeableness.
C. Openness to experience.
D. Genuineness.
E. Neuroticism.

17.6 Which personality disorder is more common in men than in women?

A. Antisocial personality disorder.
B. Borderline personality disorder.
C. Histrionic personality disorder.
D. Dependent personality disorder.
E. Schizotypal personality disorder.

17.7 Which is the only personality disorder with an age requirement and a requirement that certain childhood behaviors have continuity with adult traits?

A. Antisocial personality disorder.
B. Borderline personality disorder.
C. Avoidant personality disorder.
D. Dependent personality disorder.
E. Schizotypal personality disorder.

17.8 Does the diagnosis of a personality disorder tend to be stable over time?

A. Most personality disorders are diagnostically stable throughout life, but the severity may diminish with age.
B. Most personality disorders are diagnostically stable, and symptoms severity is stable.
C. Severity of personality disorders diminishes, and many people will make a full psychosocial recovery.
D. Severity of the personality disorder diminishes, but many people will still have some degree of interpersonal dysfunction.
E. None of the above.

17.9 Which of the following has *not* been shown to contribute to the risk of developing a personality disorder?

A. Being a victim of child abuse.
B. Witnessing domestic violence in the home.
C. Parental divorce or separation.
D. Parental absence.
E. Arrested psychosexual development.

17.10 Which personality disorder is associated with impaired smooth pursuit eye movement, impaired performance on tests of executive function, and increased ventricular-brain ratio on computed tomography?

A. Antisocial personality disorder.
B. Borderline personality disorder.
C. Schizotypal personality disorder.
D. Schizoid personality disorder.
E. Avoidant personality disorder.

17.11   Which personality disorder is associated with low resting pulse, low skin conductance, and increased amplitude on event-related potentials?

A. Antisocial personality disorder.
B. Borderline personality disorder.
C. Schizotypal personality disorder.
D. Schizoid personality disorder.
E. Avoidant personality disorder.

17.12   A 27-year-old software engineer seeks psychiatric treatment for anxiety. He has lived alone all of his adult life. Outside of work, he has no social contacts apart from a weekly phone call to his mother. He spends most of his free time playing video games, and he expresses little interest in developing more social relationships or having a romantic relationship. He does not endorse any symptoms of major depression or psychosis. He is very stiff and formal in interview and displays little emotion. What is the best diagnosis?

A. Avoidant personality disorder.
B. Schizotypal personality disorder.
C. Schizoid personality disorder.
D. Autism spectrum disorder.
E. Antisocial personality disorder.

17.13   You see a 33-year-old unemployed man in the outpatient clinic. He reports that he would like your assistance in getting disability for "anxiety." He says that for as long as he recalls, he has felt uncomfortable in social situations because he fears that other people will not understand him. He has never married and has no children. He has trouble maintaining employment due to anxiety. He sometimes thinks that magazine articles have special messages for him and may see shadows that look like people or animals. He has been trying to learn how to communicate telepathically by studying a "new age" book purchased on the Internet but has not been successful. He denies any history of auditory hallucinations and does not appear to have delusions. What is the best diagnosis?

A. Schizophrenia.
B. Schizotypal personality disorder.

C. Avoidant personality disorder.

D. Schizoid personality disorder.

E. Schizoaffective disorder.

17.14 Which of the following is *not* a trait of histrionic personality disorder?

A. Unease in situations in which one is not the center of attention.

B. Inappropriate sexually seductive or provocative behavior.

C. Rapidly shifting and shallow expression of emotions.

D. Transient, stress-related paranoid ideation or severe dissociative symptoms.

E. Self-dramatization, theatricality, and exaggerated expression of emotion.

17.15 A 26-year-old woman comes to your clinic to establish care for her mood swings that other psychiatrists have diagnosed as "bipolar disorder." She has persistent depression and severe mood swings, but she has never had a period of decreased sleep, pressured speech, or disinhibition that lasted for several days. She uses a razor blade to make small cuts on her forearms when anxious or upset but denies that she does this to kill herself. She has had several psychiatric hospitalizations for suicidal ideation, and she has overdosed multiple times. She endorses a deep fear that her loved ones will abandon her, and she has chronic feelings of emptiness. After your interview, she says that she thinks you are the best doctor she has ever had and that she has great confidence in your abilities. She speaks very poorly of her previous psychiatrist. What is the most likely diagnosis?

A. Bipolar II disorder.

B. Histrionic personality disorder.

C. Borderline personality disorder.

D. Dependent personality disorder.

E. Schizotypal personality disorder.

17.16 A 40-year-old business executive seeks treatment for depression. She reports being upset since a colleague was given a promotion that she feels was rightfully hers. Her long-term goal is to become the CEO of a major global corporation. During the session, she questions the therapist's credentials, and at one point she accuses the therapist of being envious of her superior social status. She does not return after the first session and later tells an acquaintance that it was because the therapist didn't give her the admiration that she deserves. What is the most likely diagnosis?

A. Antisocial personality disorder.
B. Borderline personality disorder.
C. Narcissistic personality disorder.
D. Dependent personality disorder.
E. Histrionic personality disorder.

17.17 Which of the following does *not* represent a recommended treatment for borderline personality disorder?

A. Dialectical behavior therapy.
B. Benzodiazepine tranquilizers for accompanying anxiety.
C. Systems Training for Emotional Predictability and Problem Solving (STEPPS).
D. Antipsychotic medications for accompanying perceptual distortions and anger dyscontrol.
E. Selective serotonin reuptake inhibitors (SSRIs) for depression.

17.18 Which of the following personality disorders is *not* a cluster C personality disorder?

A. Avoidant personality disorder.
B. Obsessive-compulsive personality disorder.
C. Histrionic personality disorder.
D. Dependent personality disorder.
E. All of the above are cluster C personality disorders.

17.19 Avoidant personality disorder can be very difficult to distinguish from which of the following disorders?

A. Social anxiety disorder.
B. Generalized anxiety disorder.
C. Panic disorder.
D. Persistent depressive disorder.
E. Autism spectrum disorder.

17.20 Ebenezer Scrooge comes to your practice seeking therapy for life dissatisfaction. He spends all of his time working even though he is very wealthy, and he is very reluctant to spend his money on basic amenities such as heating during the cold winter months. He engages in very little recreation and has very little social interaction, and he rejects his nephew's dinner invitations. He expresses rigid, controversial opinions, such as that donating to charity is wasteful given that his hard earned tax dollars finance work houses and debtors' prisons. He micromanages his sole employee, but he reserves several tasks for himself for fear that his employee is not competent to handle these necessities to his satisfaction. What is the best diagnosis for this patient?

A. Schizoid personality disorder.
B. Narcissistic personality disorder.
C. Obsessive-compulsive personality disorder.
D. Avoidant personality disorder.
E. Antisocial personality disorder.

CHAPTER 18

Psychiatric Emergencies

18.1 Aggressive behavior is associated with which of the following find-ings in the cerebrospinal fluid (CSF)?

A. Dopamine excess.
B. Norepinephrine excess.
C. Serotonin deficiency.
D. Acetylcholine deficiency.
E. Glutamine excess.

18.2 Which of the following is the single best predictor of future vio-lent behavior?

A. Threats of violence.
B. Diagnosis of a severe mental illness (e.g., schizophrenia, bipo-lar disorder).
C. Prior psychiatric hospitalization.
D. Substance abuse history.
E. History of violence.

18.3 Which of the following personality disorders is most associated with violent behavior?

A. Paranoid personality disorder.
B. Antisocial personality disorder.
C. Schizotypal personality disorder.
D. Narcissistic personality disorder.
E. Schizoid personality disorder.

18.4 Which of the following best describes the natural history of anti-social and borderline personality disorders?

A. Patients tend to act out more as they grow older.
B. Patients tend to act out less as they grow older.
C. Patients' tendency to act out does not change.
D. Patients only tend to act out less with age if they do not have a childhood history of conduct disorder.
E. Patients only tend to act out less with age if they do not have a childhood history of fire setting or cruelty to animals.

18.5. A psychiatrist is called to evaluate a patient in the emergency room whose chief complaint is homicidal ideation. The psychiatrist remains calm and speaks softly. She seats herself for the interview and allows distance between her and the patient. She is careful to always make direct eye contact and to project empathy and concern. She asks nonjudgmental questions during the interview. Which of the following behaviors displayed by the psychiatrist is *not* recommended?

A. Speaking softly.
B. Sitting during the interview, because psychiatrists should stand in order to be ready to escape.
C. Projecting empathy and concern because it can seem patronizing to a violent patient.
D. Use of direct eye contact.
E. Asking nonjudgmental questions.

18.6 You are seeing a patient with schizophrenia in the emergency room. The patient acknowledges his diagnosis and reports a worsening of symptoms. He reports he has been hearing voices that have been telling him to kill a family member, something that he does not want to do. He has been hospitalized multiple times but does not have a history of violence. The patient is pleasant and cooperative. Which of the following is the most concerning risk factor for violence?

A. Lack of insight.
B. Stated desire to hurt or kill.
C. Presence of command hallucinations.
D. Diagnosis of schizophrenia.
E. History of psychiatric hospitalization.

18.7 Which of the following combinations of medications is commonly given to calm acutely agitated patients?

A. Alprazolam and diphenhydramine.
B. Chlorpromazine and clonazepam.
C. Olanzapine and lorazepam.
D. Haloperidol and lorazepam.
E. Droperidol and alprazolam.

18.8 Fill in the blank: Suicide is the _____ leading cause of death in persons between ages 15 and 24 years.

A. First.
B. Second.
C. Third.
D. Fifth.
E. Eleventh.

18.9 Which of the following is true with regard to most people who commit suicide?

A. They usually do not tell anyone before committing suicide.
B. They may tell a friend or family member but usually do not seek medical help.
C. They usually communicate their suicidal intentions to and see physicians before they die.
D. They usually see a physician but do not usually tell their physician that they are having suicidal thoughts.
E. They usually do not have a primary care physician.

18.10 Which individual probably is at highest risk of completing suicide?

A. 25-year-old, divorced African American man.
B. 55-year-old, married white woman.
C. 60-year-old, widowed white man.
D. 19-year-old, single African American woman.
E. 40-year-old, divorced white woman.

18.11 Which of the following is *not* associated with completed suicide?

A. Depressive disorder.
B. Male sex.

C. Hopelessness.

D. Substance use disorder.

E. African American race.

18.12 Suicide is associated with which of the following in the CSF?

A. Dopamine excess.

B. Norepinephrine excess.

C. Serotonin deficiency.

D. Acetylcholine deficiency.

E. Glutamine excess.

18.13 What is the most common method used to commit suicide in the United States?

A. Overdose.

B. Cutting.

C. Hanging.

D. Firearm.

E. Jumping.

18.14 Which of the following is one of the strongest correlates of suicidal behavior, independent of psychiatric diagnosis?

A. Presence of a mental illness.

B. History of violence.

C. Recent psychiatric hospitalization.

D. Hopelessness.

E. Psychosocial stressors.

18.15 For which group of patients is suicide frequently preceded by the loss of a relationship in the past year?

A. Alcoholic persons.

B. Patients with major depressive disorder.

C. Older patients with cognitive decline.

D. Adolescents with behavior problems.

E. People with a personality disorder.

18.16 What medications are associated with lowered rates of suicide?

    A. Haloperidol.
    B. Lithium.
    C. Clozapine.
    D. Options A and B.
    E. Options B and C.

S T U D Y   G U I D E

CHAPTER 19

Legal Issues

19.1 Which of the following is a criminal and not a civil issue?

A. Determining whether to hospitalize a patient for acute homicidal ideation against his or her will.
B. Determining whether a patient with schizophrenia is capable of understanding court processes and assisting the court-appointed attorney.
C. Potential Health Insurance Portability and Accountability Act (HIPAA) violations.
D. Providing information about proposed treatments and alternatives and ensuring that the patient is capable of understanding these issues.
E. Determining whether a psychiatrist was negligent in his professional duties after abruptly terminating a doctor-patient relationship because the patient did not promptly pay a bill.

19.2 Which of the following is *not* a key criterion considered in civil commitment proceedings?

A. Mental illness.
B. Outpatient supports.
C. Dangerousness.
D. Disability.
E. Grave disability.

19.3 What level of evidence is generally required in cases of civil commitment?

A. Beyond a reasonable doubt.
B. Clear and convincing evidence.

C. Preponderance of the evidence.
D. Substantial evidence.
E. Some credible evidence.

19.4   Most states have provisions for

A. Involuntary inpatient treatment only.
B. Involuntary outpatient treatment only.
C. Both involuntary inpatient and outpatient treatment.
D. Neither involuntary nor voluntary outpatient treatment.
E. Voluntary outpatient treatment only.

19.5   In which of the following situations is it the *least* clear cut whether patient confidentiality may be broken according to our laws?

A. Reporting infectious disease such as tuberculosis or sexually transmitted infections.
B. Warning potential victims about threats made by patients.
C. Allowing access to medical charts for billing purposes.
D. Communicating with the family of a nonviolent psychiatric patient.
E. All of the above are clear cut cases in which confidentiality may be breached.

19.6   What is the most common reason psychiatrists are sued for malpractice?

A. Failure to obtain informed consent.
B. Patient suicide.
C. Alleged injuries from psychotropic medications.
D. Patient abandonment.
E. Alleged electroconvulsive therapy–related injury.

19.7   What percentage of physicians will face at least one malpractice suit at some point in their careers?

A. 10%.
B. 35%.
C. 50%.
D. 65%.
E. 80%.

19.8 According to the American Psychiatric Association, at what point does it become acceptable for a psychiatrist to have an intimate relationship with a former patient?

A. 6 months after termination of the doctor-patient relationship.
B. 1 year after termination of the doctor-patient relationship.
C. 3 years after termination of the doctor-patient relationship.
D. 10 years after termination of the doctor-patient relationship.
E. Never.

19.9 In order to be competent to stand trial, a defendant must meet all of the following criteria *except*

A. Being able to understand the nature of the charges against him or her.
B. Being able to understand the possible penalty.
C. Having been shown to have both bad behavior and blameworthy state of mind at the time of the offense.
D. Being able to understand the legal issues and procedures.
E. Being capable of working with an attorney in preparing the defense.

19.10 According to current laws, a crime occurs when

A. Illegal behavior occurs, regardless of the perpetrator's state of mind.
B. Illegal behavior occurs and the perpetrator has a blameworthy state of mind.
C. A perpetrator has a blameworthy state of mind regardless of whether illegal behavior occurs.
D. Illegal behavior occurs and the person does not have demonstrable mental illness.
E. A person with mental illness has a blameworthy state of mind.

19.11 Which of the following forms the basis of the insanity defense?

A. The *M'Naghten* standard.
B. The *Drummond* standard.
C. *Dusky v. United States*.
D. The *Tarasoff* rule.
E. The Peel Law.

19.12 A patient reveals to his psychiatrist that he plans to harm a neighbor. The psychiatrist is obligated to break confidentiality in order to protect the potential victim. How shall the psychiatrist proceed?

A. Phone the neighbor to report the threat.
B. Phone the local police.
C. Ask the patient to phone the neighbor.
D. Report the threat to the local newspaper.
E. None of the above.

19.13 A woman with a psychosis is charged with murder. During her pre-trial screening, her speech is disorganized such that she cannot engage in coherent dialogue with her attorneys. Which of the following best describes her legal situation with regard to the charges against her?

A. She is competent to stand trial but not guilty by reason of insanity.
B. She is not competent to stand trial and also not guilty by reason of insanity.
C. She is not competent to stand trial, and whether she is not guilty by reason of insanity has yet to be demonstrated.
D. She is guilty but mentally ill.
E. She has diminished capacity.

—CHAPTER 20—

Behavioral, Cognitive, and Psychodynamic Treatments

20.1 A teacher gives a child a piece of candy as a reward for answering a question correctly to encourage her students to participate more in class. This is an example of which of the following?

A. Classical conditioning.
B. Operant conditioning.
C. Behavioral activation.
D. Negative reinforcement.
E. Exposure.

20.2 The candy in the previous question functions as which of the following?

A. Behavioral activation.
B. Negative reinforcement.
C. Conditioned stimulus.
D. Positive reinforcement.
E. Unconditioned stimulus.

20.3 An earthquake occurs during a psychopharmacology lecture, frightening several psychiatry residents, although it does not cause any serious damage. In the following weeks, attendance at the psychopharmacology lectures drops significantly. The psychopharmacology lecture functions as which of the following?

A. Conditioned stimulus.
B. Unconditioned stimulus.
C. Positive reinforcement.
D. Negative reinforcement.
E. Punishment.

20.4   Gambling disorder develops through which of the following?

A. Classical conditioning.
B. Operant conditioning.
C. In vivo exposure.
D. Exposure.
E. Flooding.

20.5   A therapist has a patient visualize being in an elevator to help him overcome his fear of elevators. This is an example of which of the following?

A. Relaxation training.
B. Imaginal exposure.
C. In vivo exposure.
D. Flooding.
E. Behavioral activation.

20.6   A therapist is working with a professional musician who is suffering from depression. The patient tells the therapist that she stopped playing the guitar 2 weeks ago because it no longer brings her pleasure. She previously had been playing the guitar for a few hours daily. The therapist proposes that she begin playing the guitar again every day, in spite of her lack of interest. This is an example of which of the following?

A. Operant conditioning.
B. Imaginal exposure.
C. In vivo exposure.
D. Flooding.
E. Behavioral activation.

20.7   Which of the following is *not* part of Beck's cognitive triad of depression?

A. Negative view of oneself.
B. Negative view of relationships.

C. Negative view of the future.

D. Negative interpretation of experience.

E. More than one of the above.

20.8 Learning to correct automatic thoughts, schemas, and distortions is a key part of which kind of therapy?

A. Behavioral therapy.

B. Cognitive-behavioral therapy.

C. Interpersonal therapy.

D. Psychodynamic psychotherapy.

E. Supportive psychotherapy.

20.9 An overzealous premedical student believes that she must get a perfect score on all of her assignments to have a chance of getting in to medical school lest she be forced to spend the rest of her career working in the food service industry. This is an example of which of the following?

A. Overgeneralization.

B. Selective abstraction.

C. Dichotomous thinking.

D. Personalization.

E. Magnification and minimization.

20.10 A chess player wins three matches and loses one. He concludes that he got lucky in the three matches that he won and that he lost the other match because he is a terrible chess player. This is an example of which of the following?

A. Arbitrary inference.

B. Overgeneralization.

C. Dichotomous thinking.

D. Personalization.

E. Magnification and minimization.

20.11 A hard-working business woman arrives 30 minutes late to work because of an unexpected traffic jam caused by a car accident. She berates herself for her lack of responsibility and punctuality. This is an example of which of the following?

A. Arbitrary inference.

B. Overgeneralization.

C. Dichotomous thinking.

D. Personalization.

E. Magnification and minimization.

20.12 Which of the following represents a major difference between classical psychoanalysis and psychodynamic psychotherapy?

A. The patient is expected to do the majority of the talking.

B. One is rooted in theories developed by Freud and his followers.

C. One of the major goals is to develop insight.

D. The frequency of treatment sessions differs.

E. The neutrality of the therapist.

20.13 One of your patients is experiencing stress and anxiety that you attribute to coping with the new responsibilities that come with parenthood. Which type of psychotherapy would be especially suited to address this sort of problem?

A. Behavioral therapy.

B. Cognitive-behavioral therapy.

C. Psychodynamic psychotherapy.

D. Interpersonal therapy.

E. Supportive therapy.

20.14 Which of the following is *not* one of the four domains of interpersonal therapy?

A. Grief.

B. Interpersonal disputes.

C. Acceptance and commitment.

D. Role transitions.

E. Interpersonal deficits.

20.15 A 26-year-old woman seeks treatment of her mood instability, difficult relationships, and self-harming behaviors. She is angry and irritable and says that prior therapists have not helped. She takes fluoxetine for her depression and anxiety, but it provides little symptomatic relief. She asks if there is something else you can do for her. Which of the following programs may be beneficial to her?

A. Dialectical behavior therapy (DBT).

B. Mentalization therapy.

C. Systems Training for Emotional Predictability and Problem Solving (STEPPS).

D. Schema-focused therapy (SFT).

E. All of the above.

20.16 You are seeing a 23-year-old man with schizophrenia in your office. The patient does not have any active positive symptoms of psychosis but is very awkward in interpersonal interactions and has difficulty with everyday tasks (e.g., maintaining appropriate hygiene). Which form of therapy would be beneficial in order to improve this patient's functional status?

A. Behavioral therapy.

B. Cognitive-behavioral therapy.

C. Psychodynamic psychotherapy.

D. Interpersonal therapy.

E. Social skills training.

─CHAPTER 21─

Psychopharmacology and Electroconvulsive Therapy

21.1   What was the world's first antipsychotic?

    A. Haloperidol.
    B. Thioridazine.
    C. Fluphenazine.
    D. Chlorpromazine.
    E. Trifluoperazine.

21.2   Compared with chlorpromazine, haloperidol

    A. Has more anticholinergic side effects.
    B. Is less sedating.
    C. Causes fewer extrapyramidal side effects (EPS).
    D. Is more likely to cause orthostatic hypotension.
    E. Is associated with a much greater incidence of metabolic syndrome.

21.3   The potency of conventional antipsychotic drugs correlates most closely with which of the following?

    A. Affinity for 5-hydroxytryptamine (serotonin) type 2 receptor ($5\text{-}HT_{2A}$) receptors.
    B. Anticholinergic activity.
    C. Antihistaminic activity.
    D. Dopamine D_2 receptor affinity.
    E. Norepinephrine receptor affinity.

21.4 As a general rule, most oral antipsychotics have a half-life of about

A. 1 hour.
B. 4 hours.
C. 12 hours.
D. 1 day.
E. 5 days.

21.5 Which of the cytochrome P450 (CYP) enzymes is involved in the metabolism of antipsychotic medications?

A. 2D6.
B. 1A2.
C. 3A4.
D. 2D6, 1A2, and 3A4.
E. Metabolism does not occur because they are renally excreted.

21.6 You are following a 21-year-old man with schizophrenia on an inpatient psychiatric unit for 4 weeks. The patient continues to be floridly psychotic in spite of increasing doses of haloperidol, administered as oral tablets. His haloperidol blood level is 1 ng/mL. What does this suggest?

A. Psychotic symptoms are refractory to treatment with haloperidol.
B. The patient is a rapid metabolizer of haloperidol.
C. The patient is not swallowing the haloperidol tablets.
D. This blood level suggests laboratory error.
E. Haloperidol blood levels do not correlate with treatment response.

21.7 You are following a 21-year-old man with schizophrenia on an inpatient psychiatric unit for 6 weeks. The patient continues to be floridly psychotic in spite of increasing doses of haloperidol, administered as oral tablets. His haloperidol blood level is 15 ng/mL. What does this suggest?

A. Psychotic symptoms are refractory to treatment with haloperidol.
B. The patient is a rapid metabolizer of haloperidol.
C. The patient is not swallowing the haloperidol tablets.

D. This suggests laboratory error.

E. Haloperidol blood levels do not correlate with treatment response.

21.8 How long is an adequate trial of an antipsychotic drug?

A. 4–6 days.

B. 4–6 weeks.

C. 2–3 months.

D. 6–8 months.

E. The duration of an adequate trial depends on the specific agent.

21.9 What is the primary reason that clozapine is a second-line choice for treating psychosis?

A. Because many patients have refractory schizophrenia, clozapine is always in short supply.

B. Because clozapine can cause significant weight gain.

C. Because clozapine does not work as well as other antipsychotics for treating refractory symptoms.

D. Clozapine frequently causes agranulocytosis, making it necessary for patients to have their white blood cell counts checked regularly.

E. Because it takes 3–6 months to reach steady state.

21.10 You are seeing a 21-year-old man with schizophrenia in the outpatient clinic. His psychotic symptoms have been in remission on a moderate dose of haloperidol for the past 3 years. He has been admitted to the hospital three times for acute psychosis but has never engaged in dangerous behavior during episodes of acute psychosis. He is in school and reports that he has a good mood. The patient is interested in discontinuing antipsychotic medications, although he has tolerated the medication well. What is your recommendation?

A. "Now would be a good time for a trial without medications."

B. "We should make sure that you remain stable for another 2 years before attempting to discontinue medications."

C. "You should take the medication for the rest of your life."

D. "Let's try a new antipsychotic medication."

E. "Let's substitute a mild antidepressant for your other symptoms such as lack of motivation."

21.11 A patient with schizophrenia is admitted to an inpatient unit for acute psychosis, agitation, and violent ideation. He has had two recent (and similar admissions), and he readily admits to not taking prescribed aripiprazole tablets because he believes they are poisoned. His symptoms have responded well historically to antipsychotics that have been prescribed while he is hospitalized. Which of the following is the best long-term strategy for managing the patient's symptoms?

A. Switch to haloperidol decanoate.
B. Restart aripiprazole.
C. Switch to clozapine.
D. Switch to haloperidol.
E. Switch to risperidone.

21.12 You are seeing a 35-year-old woman with schizoaffective disorder in the outpatient clinic. The patient's psychotic symptoms have been well controlled on fluphenazine for the past several years. In interview, she displays abnormal involuntary movements of her mouth and tongue of which she is not aware. This most likely represents which of the following?

A. Pseudoparkinsonism.
B. Akathisia.
C. Tardive dyskinesia.
D. Acute dystonic reaction.
E. Anticholinergic side effect.

21.13 A 19-year-old man recently started on haloperidol for schizophrenia comes to the clinic as a walk-in requesting to be seen urgently. The patient paces in the waiting room, and in interview has trouble remaining seated in his chair and stands up frequently. He complains of severe anxiety. Which of the following best explains the patient's symptoms?

A. Akathisia.
B. New onset of generalized anxiety disorder.
C. Mania.
D. Acute dystonic reaction.
E. Tardive dyskinesia.

21.14 A 42-year-old woman presents to the emergency room complaining of muscle stiffness. Her neck is twisted to the left, and she reports that she cannot move it. She was discharged from the inpatient psychiatric unit a day earlier after receiving treatment for an acute psychosis, during which treatment with an antipsychotic agent was initiated. What is the best way to manage her symptoms?

A. Permanently discontinue the antipsychotic drug.
B. Switch to a new antipsychotic drug.
C. Administer benztropine or diphenhydramine intramuscularly.
D. Treatment with an oral benzodiazepine.
E. Psychotherapy for conversion disorder.

21.15 Which of the following is *not* an anticholinergic adverse effect of antipsychotics?

A. Diarrhea.
B. Urinary retention.
C. Blurry vision.
D. Dry mouth.
E. Exacerbation of narrow-angle glaucoma.

21.16 It has been recommended to regularly monitor body mass index (BMI), blood pressure, fasting glucose, and lipid panels for patients who are taking which of the following?

A. Haloperidol.
B. Risperidone.
C. Venlafaxine.
D. Sertraline.
E. Nortriptyline.

21.17 A 45-year-old woman who takes haloperidol for her schizophrenia is admitted to a medical unit for rigidity, high fever, and mental status changes. Laboratory tests show elevated creatinine phosphokinase and liver enzymes. What is the most important aspect of acute care for this patient?

A. Start dantrolene.
B. Start bromocriptine.
C. Start electroconvulsive therapy (ECT).
D. Stop haloperidol and provide supportive care.
E. Transfer to psychiatric unit because this is a side effect of a psychotropic agent.

21.18 You are treating a 35-year-old man for a major depressive episode and narcissistic personality disorder. He demands that he receive the most effective antidepressant available. What do you do?

    A. Prescribe levomilnacipran because it is one of the newest antidepressants.
    B. Prescribe escitalopram, because it is a standard selective serotonin reuptake inhibitor (SSRI).
    C. Prescribe venlafaxine because of its dual action in targeting norepinephrine and serotonin neurotransmission.
    D. Advise him that, for the most part, all antidepressants are equally effective.
    E. Recommend psychotherapy to address his underlying narcissism.

21.19 Which type of depression is expected to respond best to an antidepressant?

    A. Persistent depressive disorder (dysthymia).
    B. Atypical depression.
    C. Depression with comorbid hypochondriasis.
    D. Depression with comorbid somatic symptom disorder.
    E. Melancholic depression.

21.20 Which SSRI has the longest half-life?

    A. Fluoxetine.
    B. Sertraline.
    C. Citalopram.
    D. Escitalopram.
    E. Paroxetine.

21.21 Which of the following is *not* a typical SSRI adverse effect?

    A. Loose bowel movements.
    B. Anxiety.
    C. Sexual dysfunction.
    D. Nausea.
    E. Orthostatic hypotension.

21.22 You prescribe citalopram to a 28-year-old man for obsessive-compulsive disorder. At follow-up, he reports his symptoms have greatly improved, but he has developed delayed ejaculation that interferes with a new relationship. All of the following strategies have been used to address this condition *except*

A. Switch to bupropion.
B. Taking bupropion in addition to sertraline.
C. Taking cyproheptadine prior to sexual activity.
D. Taking lorazepam prior to sexual activity.
E. Taking sildenafil prior to sexual activity.

21.23 A 55-year-old woman is brought to the emergency room with an altered mental status, flushing, diaphoresis, and myoclonic jerks She was recently started on a third antidepressant agent for treatment-refractory depression. What is the most likely diagnosis?

A. Catatonia.
B. Serotonin syndrome.
C. Neuroleptic malignant syndrome (NMS).
D. SSRI discontinuation syndrome.
E. Acute dystonic reaction.

21.24 Which antidepressant is contraindicated for a 45-year-old man with epilepsy?

A. Venlafaxine.
B. Mirtazapine.
C. Trazodone.
D. Bupropion.
E. Desvenlafaxine.

21.25 Which of the following patients is a good candidate for a trial of duloxetine?

A. A 37-year-old woman with a history of multiple recent overdose attempts.
B. A 60-year-old man with chronic depression and alcoholism.
C. A 20-year-old man with depression, posttraumatic stress disorder, and insomnia.
D. A 54-year-old woman with depression partially controlled by an monoamine oxidase inhibitor (MAOI).
E. A 48-year-old man with major depression and neuropathic pain from diabetes mellitus.

21.26 Which of the following antidepressants is a good choice for a 30-year-old man with a first episode of melancholic depression with predominant features of insomnia and weight loss?

    A. Citalopram.
    B. Bupropion.
    C. Duloxetine.
    D. Mirtazapine.
    E. Venlafaxine.

21.27 Which of the following antidepressants is widely used to treat insomnia?

    A. Venlafaxine.
    B. Duloxetine.
    C. Trazodone.
    D. Phenelzine.
    E. Sertraline.

21.28 A 35-year-old man with treatment refractory depression presents to the emergency room because of a prolonged painful erection. He has been taking multiple psychotropic medications to treat his disorder, including sertraline, bupropion, buspirone, trazodone, and lithium. Which medication was most likely to have caused his condition?

    A. Sertraline.
    B. Bupropion.
    C. Buspirone.
    D. Trazodone.
    E. Lithium.

21.29 What is the mechanism of action of the new antidepressant vilazodone?

    A. It is an SSRI.
    B. It is a serotonin-norepinephrine reuptake inhibitor (SNRI).
    C. It is a dopamine D_2 receptor antagonist.
    D. It is a serotonin reuptake inhibitor and serotonin 1A ($5\text{-}HT_{1A}$) receptor partial agonist.
    E. It blocks serotonin 2 receptors and weakly inhibits serotonin reuptake.

21.30 Which of the following tricyclic antidepressants has an established therapeutic range?

A. Amitriptyline.
B. Nortriptyline.
C. Doxepin.
D. Clomipramine.
E. Protriptyline.

21.31 Why are MAOIs not more widely used to treat depression?

A. Because of the required long washout period when transitioning a patient to or from an MAOI to avoid serotonin syndrome.
B. Because when combined with foods that contain tyramine, a hypertensive crisis may result.
C. Because they are potent α-adrenergic blockers and thus cause a high frequency of orthostatic hypotension.
D. Because patients prescribed MAOIs need to carry a list of prohibited foods and wear a medical bracelet that indicates they are taking an MAOI and should carry a 10-mg tablet of nifedipine with them at all times.
E. All of the above.

21.32 Which type of antidepressant should be used in a patient with a first episode of major depression?

A. Tricyclic antidepressant.
B. SSRI.
C. SNRI.
D. MAOI.
E. Any of the above.

21.33 What is a reasonable length for an adequate trial of an antidepressant?

A. 3–5 days.
B. 3–5 weeks.
C. 1–2 months.
D. 3–4 months.
E. It depends on the agent.

21.34 A 25-year-old man with a well-established diagnosis of bipolar disorder presents to the emergency room, having been brought in by the police for disruptive behavior. He has not been sleeping for the past 3 days, and he believes he is Jesus. He is very agitated, and you feel that he is potentially dangerous. Which medication should you give him in the emergency room?

A. Lithium.
B. Valproate.
C. Lamotrigine.
D. Haloperidol.
E. Carbamazepine.

21.35 Which of the following medications has been shown to reduce suicidal behavior?

A. Valproate.
B. Lithium.
C. Carbamazepine.
D. Lamotrigine.
E. Alprazolam.

21.36 Which of the following is *not* an appropriate use of lithium?

A. Prophylaxis of manic episodes in bipolar patients.
B. Reducing the severity of manic episodes.
C. Adjunctive treatment to prevent recurrences of depression in patients with unipolar major depression.
D. Achieving rapid sedation of an acutely agitated manic patient.
E. Prophylaxis of depressive episodes in bipolar patients.

21.37 When is the best time to check a lithium blood level?

A. 8 hours after the last dose for a manic patient and 18 hours after the last dose for a euthymic patient.
B. 12 hours after the last dose.
C. 8 hours after the last dose.
D. 18 hours after the last dose.
E. Accurate lithium levels can be obtained at any time because the elimination half-life of lithium is 36 hours.

21.38 Which mood-stabilizing agent does *not* undergo mostly hepatic metabolism?

A. Valproate.
B. Lamotrigine.
C. Lithium.
D. Carbamazepine.
E. Aripiprazole.

21.39 Which mood-stabilizing agent can in rare cases cause Stevens-Johnson syndrome?

A. Valproate.
B. Lamotrigine.
C. Lithium.
D. Carbamazepine.
E. Aripiprazole.

21.40 For which of the following cases is lamotrigine monotherapy most appropriate?

A. A patient with bipolar I disorder and a history of multiple hospitalizations for mania and a history of nonresponse to lithium.
B. A patient with bipolar I disorder with a history of multiple hospitalizations for mania and a history of response to lithium.
C. A patient with bipolar I disorder who presents with irritable mania.
D. A patient with bipolar disorder with mixed mania and depression.
E. A patient with bipolar I disorder with several severe depressive episodes and infrequent manic episodes.

21.41 Which patient with bipolar disorder is a good candidate for carbamazepine therapy?

A. A patient with irritable mania who has not responded to lithium.
B. A patient in a mixed episode.
C. A patient with more than four mood episodes per year who has not responded to lithium.
D. A patient with mostly depressed episodes and mild infrequent hypomanic episodes.
E. None of the above.

21.42 Which neurotransmitter is intimately involved in the mechanism of action for benzodiazepines?

A. Glutamate.
B. Norepinephrine.
C. Gabapentin.
D. γ-Aminobutyric acid (GABA).
E. Serotonin.

21.43 Benzodiazepines are remarkably versatile drugs. These medications used to treat all of the following *except*

A. Seizure disorders.
B. Anxiety.
C. Alcohol withdrawal.
D. Sleep disorders.
E. Major depression.

21.44 Which of the following medications has a U.S. Food and Drug Administration (FDA) indication for the treatment of generalized anxiety disorder?

A. Buspirone.
B. Bupropion.
C. Alprazolam.
D. Aripiprazole.
E. None of the above.

21.45 Extrapyramidal syndromes have been treated with all of the following medications *except*

A. Propranolol.
B. Diphenhydramine.
C. Amantadine.
D. Benztropine.
E. Trazodone.

21.46 Which of the following conditions represents an absolute contraindication to administering ECT?

A. Recent myocardial infarction.
B. Unstable coronary artery disease.

C. Space-occupying brain lesions.

D. Venous thrombosis.

E. Chronically low platelet count.

21.47 A 36-year-old woman is receiving ECT for treatment of her major depression. What should she be told about possible adverse effects of the treatment?

A. She may have permanent memory loss that will be most dense around the time of treatment.

B. She will have no memory loss because the psychiatrist will use unilateral lead placement.

C. She will have permanent memory loss that will mainly involve new memories following the conclusion of the treatment.

D. She will have no memory loss because the psychiatrist will use the minimal amount of electricity needed to be therapeutic.

E. None of the above.

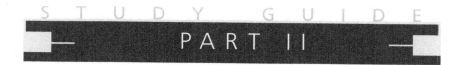

STUDY GUIDE

PART II

ANSWER GUIDE

— CHAPTER 1 —

Diagnosis and Classification

1.1 Which of the following terms is used to describe collections of symptoms that tend to co-occur and appear to have a characteristic course and outcome?

    A. Disease.
    B. Symptomatology.
    C. Syndrome.
    D. Pathophysiology.
    E. Illness.

The correct response is option C: Syndrome.

Most of the disorders or diseases diagnosed in psychiatry are *syndromes:* collections of symptoms that tend to co-occur and appear to have a characteristic course and outcome. **(p. 4)**

1.2 Which of the following is *not* a clinical reason to diagnose patients?

    A. To reduce the complexity of clinical phenomena.
    B. To provide the patient a label with which to identify.
    C. To facilitate communication between clinicians.
    D. To predict the course of illness.
    E. To determine treatment options.

The correct response is option B: To provide the patient a label with which to identify.

There are many reasons to diagnose patients. Diagnoses in psychiatry serve a variety of important purposes and are not just a "label" (option B). Making a careful diagnosis is as fundamental in psychiatry as it is in the rest of medicine. Diagnoses introduce order and structure to our thinking and reduce the complexity of clinical phenomena (option A). Diagnoses facilitate communication among clinicians (option C). The use of diagnostic categories gives clinicians a kind of "shorthand" through which they can summarize large quantities of information relatively easily. Diagnoses help to predict outcome, are often used to choose an appropriate treatment (option E), and are used to assist in the search for pathophysiology and etiology (option D). **(pp. 4–6)**

1.3 Which was the first edition of DSM to provide specific diagnostic criteria for mental disorders?

A. DSM-I.
B. DSM-II.
C. DSM-III.
D. DSM-IV.
E. DSM-5.

The correct response is option C: DSM-III.

DSM-III—published in 1980—was transformative in part because of the introduction of diagnostic criteria sets. This addition helped change the way psychiatrists and other mental health professionals go about the diagnostic process. Because of their vagueness and imprecision, the definitions in the earlier editions DSM-I (1952) and DSM-II (1968) provided brief, narrative descriptions that did not adequately fulfill many of the purposes for making a diagnosis. The authors of DSM-III agreed to formulate diagnostic criteria that would be as objective as possible to define each of the disorders and would make their decisions about defining criteria and overall organizational structure on the basis of existing research data whenever possible. **(p. 8)**

1.4 Which of the following is *not* an advantage of the DSM system?

A. It has substantially improved reliability of diagnoses.
B. It has substantially improved validity of diagnoses.
C. It has clarified the diagnostic process and history taking.

D. It has clarified and facilitated the process of differential diagnosis.

E. All of the above are advantages of the DSM system.

The correct response is option B: It has substantially improved validity of diagnoses.

DSM has improved the *reliability* (option A) of diagnoses (i.e., that clinicians will give the same patient the same diagnosis for the same symptoms). DSM has also clarified the diagnostic process, history taking, and differential diagnosis through its emphasis on diagnostic criteria (options C, D). In contrast, *validity* (option B) refers to a diagnosis's ability to predict prognosis, effective treatment, and ultimately etiology. Some have asserted that the DSM system has sacrificed validity on the altar of reliability. **(pp. 9–10)**

1.5   You are asked to evaluate a 55-year-old man on a general medical floor. You determine that he is delirious because of a hepatic encephalopathy. You learn that he drinks large quantities of distilled spirits daily and smokes one pack of cigarettes per day. Taking into account the International Classification of Diseases (ICD) and DSM rules, how would you record his diagnoses (i.e., in order of importance)?

A. Delirium (principal diagnosis), alcohol use disorder, tobacco use disorder.

B. Delirium due to hepatic encephalopathy (principal diagnosis), alcohol use disorder, tobacco use disorder.

C. Alcohol use disorder (provisional diagnosis), delirium due to hepatic encephalopathy, tobacco use disorder.

D. Hepatic encephalopathy, delirium due to hepatic encephalopathy (principal diagnosis), alcohol use disorder, tobacco use disorder.

E. Delirium due to hepatic encephalopathy, hepatic encephalopathy, alcohol use disorder, tobacco use disorder.

The correct response is option D: Hepatic encephalopathy, delirium due to hepatic encephalopathy (principal diagnosis), alcohol use disorder, tobacco use disorder.

In DSM-5, diagnoses are ranked in order of their focus of attention or treatment, listing the condition chiefly responsible for a patient's hospital stay (or outpatient clinic visit) as the *principal diagnosis* (or *reason for visit*), which may be written parenthetically after the diagnosis (e.g., "[Principal Diagnosis]"). The only exception is that—according to the arcane coding rules in the ICD system—if the mental disorder results from a medical condition, that medical condition is listed first. For example, if an outpatient with HIV disease seeks care for symptoms related to a mild neurocognitive disorder caused by the HIV, "HIV infection" is listed first, followed by "mild neurocognitive disorder due to HIV infection (reason for visit)." **(p. 13)**

1.6 You are evaluating a patient in the emergency room who you believe is likely experiencing a psychotic manic episode (bipolar I disorder with psychotic features). The patient is a poor historian, and you are not currently able to obtain collateral information to confirm the diagnosis. According to DSM, how should you document the diagnosis to reflect your uncertainty?

A. Rule out bipolar disorder, type 1.
B. Evaluate for bipolar disorder, type 1.
C. Bipolar disorder, type 1, versus psychosis not otherwise specified.
D. Bipolar disorder, type 1 (provisional).
E. Bipolar disorder, type 1.

The correct response is option D: Bipolar disorder, type 1 (provisional).

If the clinician does not have sufficient information to allow a firm diagnosis, the clinician may indicate this uncertainly by recording "(provisional)" following the diagnosis. For example, the clinical presentation may strongly suggest schizophrenia, but the patient is unable to provide sufficient history to confirm the diagnosis. **(p. 13)**

1.7 You are seeing 25-year-old woman in the outpatient clinic for a routine follow-up visit. Her major problems reported at the visit are her stormy interpersonal relationships and frequent anger outbursts. You conclude that these symptoms result from her borderline personality disorder. The patient's symptoms also meet criteria for generalized anxiety disorder, and she smokes 10 cigarettes daily. How would you record the diagnoses according to DSM-5?

A. Axis I: generalized anxiety disorder, tobacco use disorder; Axis II: borderline personality disorder (principal diagnosis).
B. Borderline personality disorder (principal diagnosis), generalized anxiety disorder, tobacco use disorder.
C. Generalized anxiety disorder, borderline personality disorder, tobacco use disorder.
D. Tobacco use disorder, borderline personality disorder, generalized anxiety disorder.
E. Borderline personality disorder (provisional), generalized anxiety disorder, tobacco use disorder.

The correct response is option B: Borderline personality disorder (principal diagnosis), generalized anxiety disorder, tobacco use disorder.

The principal diagnosis should be listed first, followed by the other diagnoses. The phrase "(principal diagnosis)" or "(reason for visit)" can be used to indicate the primary diagnosis for which the patient is seeking care. The phrase "(provisional)" is used to show that a clinician is not certain about a diagnosis, but in this vignette the clinician is confident of the diagnosis of borderline personality disorder (option E). DSM-5 no longer uses the axial system for diagnoses (option A). **(pp. 13–14)**

CHAPTER 2

Interviewing and Assessment

2.1 A psychiatrist asks a patient to recall a list of three objects ("orange, airplane, tobacco") after 5 minutes. What type of memory does this test?

A. Ultrashort-term memory.
B. Very short-term memory.
C. Short-term memory.
D. Medium-term memory.
E. Long-term memory.

The correct response is option C: Short-term memory.

Short-term memory is assessed by asking patients to recall a list of three objects after a delay of 3–5 minutes (option C). Very short-term memory, or registration, is the patient's ability to immediately recall items after he or she is told them (option B). Long-term memory is assessed by asking the patient to recall events that occurred in the more remote past (option E). Ultrashort-term and medium-term memory are not memory types (options A, D). **(p. 24)**

2.2 A psychiatrist asks a patient to tell her what the phrase "don't cry over spilled milk" means. The patient replies, "Milk isn't worth crying over because it's easy to come by." What does the patient's answer suggest?

A. Illogicality.
B. Poor abstraction.
C. Derailment.

D. Circumstantiality.

E. Poverty of content of speech.

The correct response is option B: Poor abstraction.

Proverb interpretation tests a patient's ability to think in the abstract. The patient in this example interprets the proverb literally, thus showing poor abstraction (option B). Derailment (option C) is when the patient has a pattern of spontaneous speech in which the ideas slip off the track onto another that is clearly but obliquely related or onto one completely unrelated. Illogicality (option A) refers to drawing conclusions that do not follow logically. Circumstantiality (option D) is a pattern of speech that is very indirect and delayed in reaching its goals. Poverty of content of speech (option E) is when the patient has adequate amount of speech but conveys little information. **(pp. 25–26, 39–44)**

2.3   A man believes he is preventing cancer and maximizing his health by taking an expensive but otherwise innocuous herbal supplement. If asked, he will discuss the supplement with great interest but dismisses evidence that does not confirm his beliefs. Otherwise, this interest in the supplement has no significant influence on his day-to-day life. Which of the following terms best describes the man's beliefs?

A. Overvalued ideation.

B. Delusion.

C. Poor abstraction.

D. Impaired fund of knowledge.

E. Illogicality.

The correct response is option A: Overvalued ideation.

An overvalued idea is a false belief that is held with less than a delusional intensity (option A). Delusions (option B) are more intense and fixed than overvalued ideas, and they cannot be explained on the basis of a patient's cultural background. Ability for abstraction (option C) is part of the mental status exam, and it is sometimes assessed with proverb interpretation. Nothing in the vignette suggests that the man has an impaired fund of knowledge (option D). Illogicality (option E) refers to drawing conclusions that do not follow logically. **(pp. 24–26, 31, 41)**

2.4 A patient admits to her psychiatrist that she sometimes worries that events she reads about in magazines indirectly comment on her personal life. For example, one of her favorite magazines had a recipe for banana cream pie, which made her think that somehow the editor knew this was her favorite pie. The psychiatrist asks her if she really believes this, and the patient reports that sometimes it does seem "silly." What term best describes the woman's suspicion?

A. Illogicality.
B. Persecutory delusions.
C. Delusions of reference.
D. Ideas of reference.
E. Thought broadcasting.

The correct response is option D: Ideas of reference.

Ideas of reference or *delusions of reference* are terms that describe when a patient believes that insignificant remarks, statements, or events have some special meaning for him or her. This patient is experiencing ideas of reference (option D) rather than delusions of reference (option C) because she is able to recognize that her ideas may not be true. People with persecutory delusions (option B) believe that they are being conspired against or persecuted in some way. Illogicality (option A) refers to drawing conclusions that do not follow logically. Thought broadcasting (option E) is when a patient believes that his or her thoughts are broadcast so that he or she or others can hear them. **(pp. 31–32, 34–35, 41)**

2.5 A 35-year-old woman reports to her psychiatrist that, as part of a government conspiracy, a mind control device was implanted in her brain. She believes the FBI (or possibly the CIA) is using this device to spy on her. Further, she says the device can control her body movements, making her feel like a puppet on a string. She describes how the device can remove thoughts from her brain like a vacuum cleaner while implanting thoughts that are not hers. Which of the following symptoms is *not* consistent with this patient's delusional system?

A. Delusions of passivity.
B. Thought withdrawal.
C. Thought insertion.

D. Somatic delusions.

E. Persecutory delusions.

The correct response is option D: Somatic delusions.

Somatic delusions (option D) occur when a patient believes that somehow his or her body is diseased, abnormal, or changed. This patient has a persecutory delusion (option E) that an implanted device is spying on her. The belief that the device controls her body is best described as a delusion of passivity (option A). The device can insert and delete her thoughts; this is called thought insertion (option C) and thought withdrawal (option B), respectively. **(pp. 31, 33–35)**

2.6   A psychiatrist asks a patient where she lives. She replies, "I live in Springfield. It will be spring in another couple of months, but at least this winter has been mild. The winter tends to be pretty bad in Atlanta, which is where I lived until I moved to Springfield, but birds fly south in the winter. I'd really like to go to the beach just now." What is this an example of?

A. Tangentiality.

B. Circumstantiality.

C. Incoherence.

D. Illogicality.

E. Derailment.

The correct response is option E: Derailment.

Derailment (option E) is a pattern of spontaneous speech in which the ideas slip off the track onto another that is clearly but obliquely related or onto one completely unrelated. This is not tangentiality (option A) because when a patient exhibits tangentiality, the initial answer to the question is tangential or irrelevant. Circumstantiality (option B) is speech that is indirect and delayed in reaching its goal ideas. Incoherence (option C) refers to disorganization that occurs at the level of sentences rather than at the level of the overall stream of speech. Illogicality (option D) refers to drawing conclusions that do not follow logically. **(pp. 39–41)**

2.7   A psychiatrist asks a patient if he enjoyed his own birthday party the prior week. The patient responds by laboriously describing preparations for the party and then going into minute detail about the party, including such minutiae as the order of arrival of the guests and vivid descriptions of the appetizers. Ten minutes into this story, the psychiatrist realizes that the patient never answered his question. What is this an example of?

A. Circumstantiality.
B. Pressured speech.
C. Derailment.
D. Tangentiality.
E. Distractible speech.

The correct response is option A: Circumstantiality.

Circumstantiality (option A) is speech indirect and delayed in reaching its goal ideas, which is the cardinal feature of the patient's story. This is not derailment because the content is on topic and logically connected (option C). This is not tangentiality because the patient is answering the question on topic (option D). Pressured speech is rapid and difficult to interrupt, with an increase in the overall amount of spontaneous speech. This story can be described as long-winded, but no further details are given to allow us to decide whether the speech is pressured (option B). Distractible speech (option E) occurs when the patient stops talking in the middle of a sentence or idea and changes the subject in response to a nearby stimulus. **(pp. 39–42)**

2.8   Which of the following options is a pattern of speech in which sounds rather than meaningful relationships among words appears to govern word choice?

A. Incoherence.
B. Clanging.
C. Distractible speech.
D. Pressured speech.
E. Alogia.

The correct response is option B: Clanging.

With clanging, sounds rather than meaningful relationships among words appear to govern word choice so that the intelligibility of the speech is impaired and redundant words are introduced in addition to rhyming relationships. This pattern of speech also may include punning associations, so that a word similar in sound brings in a new thought.

> *Subject:* I'm not trying to make a noise. I'm trying to make sense. If you can make sense out of nonsense, well, have fun. I'm trying to make sense out of sense. I'm not making sense [cents] anymore. I have to make dollars.

With incoherence (option A), the relationship between sounds and word choice is not necessarily present. Distractible speech (option C) occurs when the patient stops talking in the middle of a sentence or idea and changes the subject in response to a nearby stimulus. Pressured speech (option D) is rapid and difficult to interrupt. *Alogia* (option E) is a general term that describes impoverished thinking and cognition that is common in psychotic patients. **(pp. 40–43)**

2.9   A psychiatrist is interviewing a manic patient. The patient speaks very rapidly, and it is very difficult for the psychiatrist to get a word in. The patient is unable to adequately answer many routine questions because he is distracted by objects in the room such as chairs, the psychiatrist's neck tie, and the clock on the wall. Which of the following options best describes the patient's speech?

A. Pressured speech.
B. Distractible speech.
C. Both pressured speech and distracted speech.
D. Catatonic excitement.
E. Circumstantiality.

The correct response is option C: Both pressured speech and distractible speech.

The patient's speech is both pressured and distracted because it is rapid and difficult to interrupt, and he is unable to answer questions adequately because he is distracted by environmental stimuli (option C).

With pressured speech, the patient has an increase in the amount of spontaneous speech compared with what is considered ordinary or socially customary. The patient talks rapidly and is difficult to interrupt (option A). Pressured speech is often seen in mania but can be found in other syndromes as well. Some sentences may be left uncompleted because of eagerness to get on to a new idea. Speech tends to be loud and emphatic. With distracted speech, however, the patient may stop talking in the middle of a sentence or idea and changes the subject in response to a nearby stimulus, such as an object on a desk, the interviewer's clothing or appearance, and so forth (option B).

> *Subject:* Then I left San Francisco and moved to...where did you get that tie? It looks like it's left over from the '50s. I like the warm weather in San Diego. Is that a conch shell on your desk? Have you ever gone scuba diving?

Catatonic excitement (option D) is when a patient has purposeless and stereotyped excited motor activity not influenced by external stimuli. Circumstantiality (option E) is speech that is indirect and delayed in reaching its goal ideas. **(pp. 41–43)**

2.10   In response to a routine question, a patient begins to answer appropriately, but stops talking mid-sentence, and stares off into space for 15 seconds. She then asks the interviewer to repeat the question. What does this exemplify?

A. Poverty of speech.
B. Poverty of content of speech.
C. Circumstantiality.
D. Perseveration.
E. Thought blocking.

The correct response is option E: Thought blocking.

Thought blocking (option E) describes when a patient's train of speech is interrupted before completion. Poverty of speech (option A) is a restricted amount of spontaneous speech so that replies to questions tend to be brief, concrete, and unelaborated. Poverty of content of speech (option B) is when speech is adequate in amount but conveys little information. Perseveration (option D) is persistent repetition of words, ideas, or phrases by the patient. Circumstantiality (option C) is speech that is indirect and delayed in reaching its goal ideas. **(pp. 41, 43–45)**

2.11   A psychiatrist notes that a patient is very slow to answer questions and that his speech and body movements are slow. What is the correct term for this symptom?

A. Depression.
B. Psychomotor retardation.
C. Psychomotor agitation.
D. Thought blocking.
E. Alogia.

The correct response is option B: Psychomotor retardation.

Psychomotor retardation (option B) occurs when a patient feels slowed down and experiences great difficulty moving. Psychomotor slowing is often found in depression, but it is only one symptom of the depressive syndrome (option A). Psychomotor agitation (option C) is exhibited when the patient is unable to sit still and has a need to keep moving. Thought blocking (option D) describes when patients lose track of their thoughts prior to their completion. Alogia (option E) refers to the impoverished thinking and cognition that often occurs in patients with schizophrenia. **(pp. 43–44, 52)**

— CHAPTER 3 —

Neurobiology and Genetics of Mental Illness

3.1 Which of the following is *not* a primary function of the prefrontal system?

A. High-order abstract thought.
B. Creative problem solving.
C. Fear processing.
D. Temporal sequencing of behavior.
E. Moral judgment.

The correct response is option C: Fear processing.

Fear processing is associated with the limbic system, especially the amygdala (option C). Options A, B, D, and E are primary functions of the prefrontal system. This huge association region in the brain integrates input from much of the neocortex, limbic regions, hypothalamic and brainstem regions, and (via the thalamus) most of the rest of the brain. Its high degree of development in human beings suggests that it may mediate a variety of specifically human functions often referred to as *executive functions,* such as high-order abstract thought, creative problem solving, and the temporal sequencing of behavior. Lesion and trauma studies, supplemented by experimental studies in nonhuman primates, have substantially added to this view of the functions of the prefrontal cortex. It is now clear that the prefrontal cortex mediates a large variety of functions, including attention and perception, moral judgment, temporal integration, and affect and emotion. **(pp. 59–61)**

3.2   Which of the following areas of the brain have a high concentra-
        tion of dopamine D_2 receptors and may be important sites for an-
        tipsychotic drug action?

        A. Locus coeruleus.
        B. Caudate and putamen.
        C. Raphe nuclei.
        D. Nucleus basalis.
        E. None of the above.

        The correct response is option B: Caudate and putamen.

        The basal ganglia are relevant to psychiatry because of their chemi-
        cal anatomy. The caudate and putamen contain a very high concen-
        tration of dopamine receptors (option B), particularly D_2 receptors.
        The efficacy of antipsychotic medications is highly correlated
        with their ability to block D_2 receptors. Because D_2 receptors
        have a very high density in these regions, the caudate and puta-
        men may be important sites for antipsychotic drug action. The
        norepinephrine system arises in the locus coeruleus (option A),
        while the serotonin system arises in the raphe nuclei (option C).
        The cholinergic system arises in the nucleus basalis (option D).
        (p. 64)

3.3   Which part of the brain is dedicated to speech production?

        A. Broca's area.
        B. Nucleus basalis.
        C. Angular gyrus.
        D. Wernicke's area.
        E. Amygdala.

        The correct response is option A: Broca's area.

        Within the left hemisphere, there are two major language regions
        as well as some subsidiary ones. Broca's area is the region dedi-
        cated to the production of speech (option A). It contains informa-
        tion about the syntactical structure of language, provides the
        "little words" such as prepositions that tie the fabric of language
        together, and is the generator for fluent speech. Lesions to Broca's
        area, which occur in stroke victims, lead to halting, stammering,
        and ungrammatical speech. Wernicke's area (option D) is often re-

ferred to as the "auditory association cortex." It encodes the information that permits us to "understand" the sounds expressed in speech. The perception of sound waves, which encode speech, occurs through transducers in the ear that convert the information to neural signals. The signals are received in the auditory cortex, but the meaning of the specific signals cannot be understood (i.e., perceived as constituting words with specific meanings—as opposed, for example, to the wordless music of a symphony) without being compared with "templates" in Wernicke's area. The angular gyrus is a visual association cortex that contains the information or templates that permit us to recognize language presented in visual form (option C). The nucleus basalis (option B) lies in the ventral and medial regions of the globus pallidus and helps mediate memory. The amygdala (option E) forms part of the limbic system and is implicated in a variety of anxiety disorders. **(pp. 65–66)**

3.4 The nucleus accumbens is a key part of which functional system in the brain?

A. Executive system.
B. Limbic system.
C. Memory system.
D. Attention system.
E. Reward system.

The correct response is option E: Reward system.

The nucleus accumbens is a key part of the reward system of the brain. Other areas involved in reward processing are the ventral tegmental area, the prefrontal cortex, the amygdala, and the hippocampus. The reward system is relevant to many types of psychiatric disorders. It is often said that substance abuse develops when exposure to a drug such as cocaine "highjacks the brain reward system" by inducing an intense experience of pleasure that stimulates craving and repeated drug-seeking behavior. This system has been implicated in all types of dependence on both illegal (e.g., amphetamines, opiates) and legal (e.g., nicotine, alcohol) substances. It is also thought to provide the basis for other types of pleasure-seeking or addictive behaviors and their consequences, such as gambling disorder or compulsive overeating. **(p. 68)**

3.5   What is the primary neurotransmitter in the brain reward system, which is also associated with adventuresome and exploratory behaviors?

A. Dopamine.
B. Norepinephrine.
C. γ-Aminobutyric acid (GABA).
D. Serotonin.
E. Glutamate.

The correct response is option A: Dopamine.

Dopamine is the primary neurotransmitter in the brain reward system and is associated with adventuresome and exploratory behavior (option A). Serotonin (option D) plays a role in modulating mood, anxiety, and aggressive behavior. Norepinephrine (option B) is thought to play a role in mood disorders. Glutamate (option E) is an excitatory neurotransmitter that plays a role in learning and memory. GABA (option C) is important to understanding anxiety disorders because many anxiolytics such as diazepam act as GABA agonists. **(pp. 68–72, 75)**

3.6   Where does the brain's norepinephrine system originate?

A. Raphe nuclei.
B. Hypothalamus.
C. Ventral tegmental area.
D. Locus coeruleus.
E. Nucleus accumbens.

The correct response is option D: Locus coeruleus.

The norepinephrine system originates in the locus coeruleus (option D). The serotonin system originates in the raphe nuclei (option A), and the ventral tegmental area (option C) gives rise to the dopamine system. The nucleus accumbens (option E) is important in the reward system. The hypothalamus (option B) receives projections from the locus coeruleus and raphe nuclei, but it is not the site of origin of the norepinephrine or serotonergic system. **(pp. 68–72)**

3.7   Which of the following nuclei in the brain contains the cell bodies of an important group of acetylcholine neurons?

A. Nucleus basalis.
B. Locus coeruleus.
C. Raphe nuclei.
D. Substantia nigra.
E. Caudate nucleus.

The correct response is option A: Nucleus basalis.

The nucleus basalis contains the cell bodies of an important group of cholinergic neurons (option A). The locus coeruleus (option B) gives rise to the norepinephrine system, and the raphe nuclei (option C) give rise to the serotonin system. The substantia nigra (option D) contains dopaminergic neurons that have some projections to the caudate nucleus (option E). **(pp. 69–74)**

3.8   Which neurotransmitter provides inhibitory modulation to the globus pallidus, which if lost, will result in the choreiform movements of Huntington's disease?

A. Dopamine.
B. Serotonin.
C. Acetylcholine.
D. Glutamate.
E. GABA.

The correct response is option E: GABA.

GABA provides inhibitory modulation of the globus pallidus, which if lost, will result in the choreiform movements of Huntington's disease (option E). Aberrancy of dopaminergic transmission also plays a key role in the pathology of Huntington's disease (option A). Glutamate (option D) is an excitatory rather than an inhibitory neurotransmitter. Serotonin and acetylcholine (options B, C) do not play primary roles in this process. **(pp. 74–75)**

3.9   Family studies of mental illness have shown that most major mental illnesses "run in families." Which of the following is *not* an essential element of a family study?

A. Identifying people with the disorder of interest (e.g., schizophrenia).
B. Identifying people who can serve as control subjects.
C. Interviewing first-degree relatives of ill persons and control subjects.
D. Comparing rates of the disorder of interest in relatives of those with the mental illness in question and relatives of control subjects.
E. Showing that the illness in question is inherited.

The correct response is option E: Showing that the illness in question is inherited.

Family studies examine the pattern of aggregation within a family, beginning with the identification of a proband (or index case) who has a particular disorder of interest, such as bipolar disorder or schizophrenia (option A). Thereafter, all available first-degree relatives (parents, siblings, children) are also evaluated using structured interviews and diagnostic criteria (option C). The prevalence of the specific disorder under investigation is compared with the prevalence in a carefully selected control group (option B). If an increased rate of the specific mental illness under study is observed in the first-degree relatives of the probands as compared with the first-degree relatives of the control subjects, then these results suggest that a disorder is familial and possibly genetic (option D). These studies cannot exclude the possibility that the disorder has prominent nongenetic causes and therefore cannot determine if a disorder is inherited (option E). Disorders can also run in families because of learned behavior, role modeling, or predisposing social environments. **(pp. 76–77)**

3.10 Which type of study applies statistical analyses to large databases containing DNA from thousands of individuals affected by specific disorders?

A. Linkage study.
B. Candidate gene study.
C. Genome-wide association study.
D. Copy number variant survey.
E. Microarray analysis.

The correct response is option C: Genome-wide association study.

Genome-wide association studies apply statistical analyses to large databases containing DNA from thousands of individuals affected by specific disorders (option C). Linkage studies attempt to correlate diseases with specific sites on chromosomes (option A). Candidate gene studies typically begin with hypothesis-driven selection of a candidate gene (option B), for example, vulnerability genes for schizophrenia such as the brain-derived neurotrophic factor (BDNF) gene and the dysbindin-1 gene *DTNBP1*. Microarray analysis is a technique used in molecular biology that is not discussed in the text (option E). Copy number variants have the potential to confer disease liability, but copy number variant survey is not a type of research study (option D). **(pp. 79–81)**

— CHAPTER 4 —

Neurodevelopmental (Child) Disorders

4.1   What is the standard test used to assess the intelligence of children between 6 and 16 years of age?

A. Stanford-Binet Intelligence Scale.
B. Wechsler Intelligence Scale for Children.
C. Peabody Picture Vocabulary Test.
D. Kaufman ABC.
E. Wechsler Preschool and Primary Scale of Intelligence.

The correct response is option B: Wechsler Intelligence Scale for Children.

The Wechsler Intelligence Scale for Children (WISC-IV) is the standard instrument for assessing the intelligence of school-age children between the ages 6 and 16 years (option B). Younger children can be assessed with the Kaufman ABC (option D) or Wechsler Preschool and Primary Scale of Intelligence (option E). The WISC-IV consists of a group of 10 core subtests that assess a variety of cognitive functions (e.g., vocabulary, comprehension, block design, matrix reasoning, digit span, symbol search). These are used to generate a full-scale IQ, verbal and performance IQs, and four composite scores known as indices (verbal comprehension, perceptual organization, processing speed, and working memory). The Stanford-Binet Intelligence Scale (option A) is one of the oldest scales and can be used for some younger children. The Peabody Picture Vocabulary Test (option C) can be used to assess vocabulary and scholastic aptitude. The test uses pictures to provide a measure of oral language comprehension, from which verbal intelligence can be inferred. In general, IQ based on the Peabody or other similar tests tends to be an overestimate. **(pp. 91–93)**

4.2   What is the standard deviation of IQ on the WISC-IV?

A. 100.
B. 85.
C. 15.
D. 25.
E. 115.

The correct response is option C: 15.

Examining the scores on individual WISC-IV subtests gives clinicians a sense of the child's overall intellectual skills and weaknesses. The test is scaled to have a mean of 100 and a standard deviation of 15. Sixty-seven percent of children have IQs that fall between 85 and 115, whereas 95% have IQs that fall between 70 and 130. **(p. 92)**

4.3   Which of the following scales can be used to assess for attention-deficit/hyperactivity disorder (ADHD)?

A. Benton Visual Retention Test.
B. Vineland Adaptive Behavior Scale.
C. Thematic Apperception Test.
D. Conners Teacher Rating Scale—Revised.
E. Bender-Gestalt.

The correct response is option D: Conners Teacher Rating Scale—Revised.

Conners Teacher Rating Scale—Revised can be used by teachers to assess behaviors associated with ADHD in the classroom (option D). The Vineland Adaptive Behavior Scale (option B) measures adaptive skills in children. The Benton Visual Retention Test (option A) and the Bender-Gestalt (option E) assess perceptual-motor skills. The Thematic Apperception Test (option C) is a personality assessment. **(pp. 93–94)**

4.4   What is the most common heritable cause of intellectual disability?

A. Down syndrome.
B. Fragile X.
C. Tay-Sachs.
D. Prader-Willi syndrome.
E. Williams syndrome.

The correct response is option B: Fragile X.

Fragile X is the most common heritable cause of intellectual disability (option B). Down syndrome is the most common chromosomal cause (option A). Options C–E are less common causes of intellectual disability. **(pp. 98–99)**

4.5   A 25-year-old man with intellectual disability has lived in a group home all of his adult life. He can read his name and a few other words. He is able to take care of his activities of daily living such as bathing and other personal hygiene tasks and doing laundry. He was in special education classes throughout school. What is the probable severity of his intellectual disability?

A. Mild.
B. Moderate.
C. Severe.
D. Profound.
E. Unable to estimate.

The correct response is option B: Moderate.

This patient's level of impairment is consistent with moderate intellectual disability. Patients with mild intellectual disability are capable of living in the community, working, reading, writing, and doing basic arithmetic. Patients with severe and profound intellectual disability generally require an institutionalized care setting. **(p. 97)**

4.6   What is the DSM-5 diagnosis for a child who stutters?

A. Language disorder.
B. Speech sound disorder.
C. Childhood-onset fluency disorder.

D. Social (pragmatic) communication disorder.

E. Autism spectrum disorder.

The correct response is option C: Childhood-onset fluency disorder.

Childhood-onset fluency disorder is the correct diagnosis for children who stutter (option C). Language disorder (option A) is a deficit in comprehension and or production of language. Speech sound disorder (option B) is a disorder of speech production that accounts for phenomena such as articulation errors. Children who have difficulty tailoring their communication appropriately to the social context are diagnosed with social (pragmatic) communication disorder (option D). Patients with autism spectrum disorder (option E) have difficulties with social communication and display a pattern of restricted, stereotyped interests. **(pp. 100–102)**

4.7 An 8-year-old boy is brought to a child psychiatrist for an evaluation. His parents report that he is socially awkward and has trouble making friends. His grades are very good. The boy is polite but overly formal in conversation. He avoids eye contact. His parents report that he sticks to a rigid routine at home and has an unusually intense interest in U.S. presidents and can name all of them in correct order. When this is brought up, the child begins a lengthy discourse on them. What is the best diagnosis?

A. Language disorder.

B. Speech sound disorder.

C. Childhood-onset fluency disorder.

D. Social (pragmatic) communication disorder.

E. Autism spectrum disorder.

The correct response is option E: Autism spectrum disorder.

Patients with autism spectrum disorder have difficulties with social communication and display a pattern of restricted, stereotyped interests (option E). Language disorder (option A) is a deficit in comprehension and or production of language. Speech sound disorder (option B) is a disorder of speech production that accounts for phenomena such as articulation errors. Social (pragmatic) communication disorder (option D) is a diagnosis used in children who have difficulty tailoring their communication appropriately to the social context. Childhood-onset fluency disorder (option C) is a diagnosis for children who stutter. **(pp. 102–107)**

4.8 How does treatment with stimulant medications affect risk of substance abuse in persons diagnosed with ADHD?

A. Use of stimulant medications increases the risk of any substance abuse.
B. Use of stimulant medications decreases the risk of any substance abuse.
C. Use of stimulant medications does not affect the risk of substance abuse.
D. Use of stimulant medications is associated with a worse long-term outcome.
E. Use of stimulant medications increases the risk for abuse of stimulant medications only.

The correct response is option B: Use of stimulant medications decreases the risk of any substance abuse.

Research has shown that using stimulant medications to treat ADHD decreases the patient's risk of substance abuse. Treating the disorder brings symptomatic relief and can lead to a better long-term outcome. **(p. 112)**

4.9 What is the prevalence of ADHD in children?

A. 1%–2%.
B. 5%.
C. 10%.
D. 20%.
E. >30%.

The correct response is option B: 5%.

The prevalence of ADHD in children is around 5%. **(p. 112)**

4.10 A 9-year-old boy is brought to his pediatrician by his parents, who are concerned about the possibility of ADHD. A written report from his teacher says that he is frequently in trouble for fighting with other children and that he refuses to obey classroom rules. He frequently steals small items from his peers and the school cafeteria. He also talks out of turn and has trouble staying in his seat. His parents report that he has lots of energy and that he "bounces off the walls" at home. He talks back to his parents. Which of the following symptoms in this case is suggestive of ADHD?

A. Fighting with other children.
B. Refusal to obey classroom rules.
C. Stealing.
D. Talking back to parents.
E. Difficulty staying in his seat.

The correct response is option E: Difficulty staying in his seat.

Having trouble staying seated is suggestive of ADHD (option E). Fighting and stealing (options A, C) suggest a diagnosis of conduct disorder. Refusing to obey rules and talking back to parents (options B, D) are suggestive of either conduct disorder or oppositional defiant disorder. These disorders are often comorbid. **(pp. 107–114)**

4.11 Which of the following medications is a first-line treatment for ADHD?

A. Guanfacine.
B. Methylphenidate.
C. Clonidine.
D. Bupropion.
E. Atomoxetine.

The correct response is option B: Methylphenidate.

Methylphenidate is usually the first-line treatment for ADHD (option B), followed by dextroamphetamine. Atomoxetine (option E), an α_2 agonist (e.g., clonidine, guanfacine [options A, C]), imipramine, or bupropion (option D) are second-line treatments. **(p. 113)**

4.12 Which of the following is *not* a common side effect of the stimulant medications commonly used to treat ADHD?

A. Weight gain.
B. Insomnia.

C. Stomach upset.

D. Irritability.

E. Appetite suppression.

The correct response is option A: Weight gain.

Weight loss, not weight gain (option A), is a common side effect of stimulants. For this reason, weight should be monitored in children prescribed stimulants. Options B–E are common side effects of stimulants. **(pp. 113–114)**

4.13   A 9-year-old boy of average intelligence is making satisfactory grades in all subjects in school with the exception of math, which he is failing. His Iowa Test of Basic Skills score confirms satisfactory performance on all subjects except math, which is considerably lower than average. He sometimes shows irritation and frustration in the classroom during math class, but his behavior is otherwise unremarkable. His parents do not have concerns about his mood or behavior at home. What is the most beneficial intervention for this child?

A. Remedial instruction in math and instruction in compensatory learning strategies.

B. Start methylphenidate.

C. Start fluoxetine.

D. Start atomoxetine.

E. Referral for cognitive-behavioral therapy.

The correct response is option A: Remedial instruction in math and instruction in compensatory learning strategies.

This child has a specific learning disorder. The standard treatment for a specific learning disorder is to provide remedial instruction in the area of weakness and also in learning compensatory strategies (option A). Medications and cognitive-behavioral therapy (options B–D) have no role in its treatment. **(pp. 115–116)**

4.14   Which of the following is *not* considered a stereotypic movement when considering the diagnosis of stereotypic movement disorder?

A. Head banging.

B. Rocking.

C. Hitting one's own body.

D. Nonrhythmic, jerky movements of the neck.

E. Hand waving.

The correct response is option D: Nonrhythmic, jerky movements of the neck.

Nonrhythmic jerky movements of the neck (option D) are better classified as tics. Options A–C and E can be types of stereotypic movements. **(pp. 116–117)**

4.15 How is the diagnosis of Tourette's disorder different from a persistent motor or vocal tic disorder?

A. Patients with Tourette's disorder have coprolalia (offensive vocal tics).

B. Tics in Tourette's disorder are of longer duration than tics that occur in motor or vocal tic disorder.

C. Patients with Tourette's disorder have both motor and vocal tics.

D. Tourette's disorder is associated with streptococcal infection.

E. Tourette's disorder has high comorbidity with obsessive-compulsive disorder.

The correct response is option C: Patients with Tourette's disorder have both motor and vocal tics.

Patients with Tourette's disorder have both motor and vocal tics, which differentiates this disorder from chronic motor or vocal tic disorder (option C), in which the patients have only motor or vocal tics but not both. The vocal tics accompanying Tourette's disorder can be somewhat socially offensive (option A). Tics tend to be of similar duration regardless of specific diagnosis (option B). Some cases of Tourette's disorder are associated with streptococcal infection (option D) and may have comorbidity with obsessive-compulsive disorder (option E), but these features do not need to be present for diagnosis. **(pp. 117–119)**

4.16 Which of the following medications are U.S. Food and Drug Administration (FDA) approved for treatment of pediatric depression?

A. Fluoxetine and escitalopram.
B. Citalopram and paroxetine.
C. Venlafaxine and nefazodone.
D. Sertraline and citalopram.
E. Escitalopram and citalopram.

The correct response is option A: Fluoxetine and escitalopram.

Fluoxetine and escitalopram are FDA approved for the treatment of pediatric depression. **(p. 120)**

— CHAPTER 5 —

Schizophrenia Spectrum and Other Psychotic Disorders

5.1 Which of the following statements *mischaracterizes* schizophrenia?

A. Patients have a "split" personality.
B. Patients have disability in their capacity to think clearly.
C. Patients have disability in their capacity to experience normal emotions.
D. Patients typically develop symptoms in early adulthood.
E. Patients often develop bizarre hallucinations and delusions.

The correct response is option A: Patients have a "split" personality.

Patients with schizophrenia do not have a split personality (option A) or multiple personalities. Options B–E are generally true of schizophrenia. **(p. 125)**

5.2 You have been seeing a 45-year-old man in the outpatient clinic for "stress." He relates his stress to what he believes was a conspiracy by former coworkers to get him fired from his previous job by "arranging" work-related incidents that would reflect poorly on him. He has threatened to sue, but because of lack of evidence, no lawyer has agreed to take his case. As his psychiatrist, you find yourself unable to get him to talk about other issues. He has never had hallucinations, disorganized behavior, mania, or frank depression. What is the most likely diagnosis?

A. Schizophrenia.
B. Schizoaffective disorder.
C. Schizophreniform disorder.
D. Delusional disorder.
E. Bipolar I disorder.

The correct response is option D: Delusional disorder.

People with a delusional disorder have delusions accompanied by minimal (or no) hallucinations, and their behavior apart from the delusion or its ramifications is not markedly bizarre or odd (option D). These individuals are often described as overtalkative and circumstantial, particularly when discussing their delusions. They do not exhibit other symptoms of schizophrenia (option A) and schizophreniform disorder (option C) such as disorganized thinking or behavior. Schizoaffective disorder (option B) and bipolar disorder (option E) are not likely given the absence of a mood disturbance. **(pp. 126–130)**

5.3   At what age do women typically develop schizophrenia?

A. 13–18 years.
B. 18–25 years.
C. 21–30 years.
D. 35–50 years.
E. >50 years.

The correct response is option C: 21–30 years.

Women typically develop symptoms between ages 21 and 30 years. Men typically develop symptoms between ages 18 and 25. **(p. 135)**

5.4   Which of the following is an example of a "first-rank" symptom of schizophrenia as identified by psychiatrist Kurt Schneider?

A. The patient believes thoughts are being inserted into his or her mind.
B. The patient believes the government is spying on him or her.
C. The patient believes that his or her masturbation has led to insanity.

D. The patient believes the somatic delusion that his or her heart has stopped beating.

E. The patient experiences the tactile hallucination that insects are crawling under his or her skin.

The correct response is option A: The patient believes thoughts are being inserted into his or her mind.

Schneider, a German psychiatrist working in the early twentieth century, argued that certain types of hallucinations and delusions were of the "first rank," meaning that they are especially characteristic of schizophrenia. Examples include delusions of being forced to do things against one's will or that thoughts are being withdrawn from or inserted into one's mind (option A). These symptoms all reflect a patient's confusion about the loss of boundaries between himself or herself and the external world. Options B–D are examples of delusions commonly seen in persons with psychosis but are not examples of "first-rank" delusions. Option E refers to formication, which is a hallucination in which the person feels that insects are crawling under his or her skin, and is also not considered a first-rank symptom. **(pp. 136–137)**

5.5   You are evaluating a 30-year-old woman with schizophrenia on a psychiatric inpatient unit. She reports that she has died and has gone to heaven to be with Jesus. She will not accept any evidence to the contrary. What type of delusion is this?

A. Persecutory delusion.
B. Grandiose delusion.
C. Nihilistic delusion.
D. Somatic delusion.
E. Religious delusion.

The correct response is option C: Nihilistic delusion.

Patients with nihilistic delusions believe that they are dead or dying (option C) or that they or the world does not exist. Grandiose delusions (option B) involve the patient having special powers or eminence. Persecutory delusions (option A) have as their theme being spied on or plotted against. Somatic delusions (option D) involve bodily functions ("my heart has stopped beating"). Religious delusions (option E) tend to concern having a special relationship with a higher power or a special religious mission. **(Table 5–2 [Varied content in delusions], p. 137)**

5.6 Which phase of schizophrenia is characterized by subtle behavior changes that include social withdrawal, work impairment, blunting of emotion, avolition, and odd ideas and behavior?

A. Prodromal phase.
B. Active phase.
C. Residual phase.
D. Cataleptic phase.
E. Schizoaffective phase.

The correct response is option A: Prodromal phase.

The prodromal phase of schizophrenia is characterized by subtle behavior changes that include social withdrawal, work impairment, blunting of emotion, avolition, and odd ideas and behavior (option A). The active phase is characterized by hallucinations, delusions, or disorganized speech and behavior (option B). The residual phase is characterized by role impairment, negative symptoms, and attenuated positive symptoms (option C). The terms *cataleptic* and *schizoaffective* (options D, E) do not refer to typical phases of schizophrenia. **(Table 5–4 [Typical stages of schizophrenia], p. 142)**

5.7 You are treating a patient with schizophrenia on an inpatient unit. The patient has displayed disorganized behavior throughout hospitalization. One day at morning rounds, the patient mimics your hand gestures without reason. What is the term for this behavior?

A. Echolalia.
B. Echopraxia.
C. Catalepsy.
D. Negativism.
E. Stereotypy.

The correct response is option B: Echopraxia.

Echopraxia is a type of disorganized behavior in which a patient will mimic an examiner's movements or mannerisms (option B).

Echolalia is manifested when a patient repeats things that are said in his or her presence (option A). Catalepsy refers to a rigid body state with waxy flexibility (option C). When a patient refuses to perform simple requests for no apparent reason (option D), this is called negativism. Stereotypy (option E) refers to purposeless repetitive movements such as rocking back and forth. **(pp. 139, 142)**

5.8   A 20-year-old man with schizophrenia comes to your clinic for a scheduled follow-up visit, accompanied by his mother, with whom he lives. His disorder is well controlled with low-dose antipsychotic medication. He reports mild auditory hallucinations but says they do not bother him. His mother is concerned that the patient is inactive much of the day and must be prompted to groom himself. He prefers to watch TV all day without engaging in any other activities. The patient shows some affective blunting but denies depressed mood. He reports restful sleep and has a healthy appetite. He tolerates his medication without noticeable adverse effects and says he feels "pretty good" about his current situation. How should you address the mother's concerns?

A. Prescribe a stimulant to increase his energy.
B. Prescribe an antidepressant to treat his negative symptoms.
C. Reassess the patient for schizoaffective disorder and consider adding a mood stabilizer.
D. Reduce the dose of the antipsychotic medication.
E. Provide psychoeducation to the patient's mother.

The correct response is option E: Provide psychoeducation to the patient's mother.

Avolition is a common negative symptom of schizophrenia, and there are no standardized effective guidelines for addressing this issue medically. As such, it is wise to educate the family about schizophrenia and its many symptoms (option E), including amotivation. Stimulants could lead to a worsening of his psychosis (option A). Antidepressants are not clearly indicated because the patient denies depression and has no depressive symptoms (option B). Reducing the dose of the antipsychotic medication (option D) could lead to relapse of positive symptoms, and it is not clear that this would help the patient with his negative symptoms. Furthermore, he is on a low dose of an antipsychotic and does not report adverse effects. The patient has not had a clear-cut depressive or manic episode, so there is no reason to diagnose schizoaffective disorder (option C). **(pp. 138, 143, 148–149)**

5.9   A 24-year-old woman is admitted to an inpatient psychiatric unit for acute psychosis. She endorses auditory hallucinations and persecutory delusions and has an inappropriate affect. She has no previous episodes, she has not been abusing substances, and medical workup does not show a clear etiology for her symptoms. She has not shown clear symptoms of major depression or of mania. At this point, her total duration of illness is 2 weeks. What is the best diagnosis at this time?

A. Schizophrenia.
B. Schizoaffective disorder.
C. Schizophreniform disorder.
D. Brief psychotic disorder.
E. Bipolar disorder.

The correct response is option D: Brief psychotic disorder.

Because the total duration of illness is less than 1 month, the appropriate diagnosis is brief psychotic disorder (option D). Patients with a total duration of illness from 1 month to 6 months should be diagnosed with schizophreniform disorder (option C). Patients whose total duration of illness exceeds 6 months should be diagnosed with schizophrenia (option A). Schizoaffective disorder (option B) and bipolar disorder (option E) are not appropriate diagnoses because there is no evidence of a mood disturbance. **(pp. 131–133)**

5.10   Postpartum psychosis is a subtype of which DSM-5 psychotic disorder?

A. Schizophrenia.
B. Schizoaffective disorder.
C. Schizophreniform disorder.
D. Brief psychotic disorder.
E. Bipolar disorder.

The correct response is option D: Brief psychotic disorder.

According to DSM-5, postpartum psychosis is a subtype of brief psychotic disorder (option D), and it should be written as brief psychotic disorder with postpartum onset. Postpartum psychosis is not a subtype of options A–C or E. **(pp. 131–132)**

5.11   A 24-year-old woman is admitted to an inpatient psychiatric unit for acute psychosis in the setting of medication noncompliance. She reports auditory hallucinations and persecutory delusions and has an inappropriate affect. She has no previous episodes, she has not been abusing substances, and medical workup does not show a clear etiology of her symptoms. She has not shown clear symptoms of major depression or of mania. This episode has been going on for the past 2 weeks. Two months previously, she had her first psychotic episode, which lasted for 3 weeks, but she went into remission with antipsychotic therapy. What is the best diagnosis?

A. Schizophrenia.
B. Schizoaffective disorder.
C. Schizophreniform disorder.
D. Brief psychotic disorder.
E. Bipolar disorder.

The correct response is option C: Schizophreniform disorder.

A diagnosis of schizophreniform disorder is given to patients who have psychotic symptoms suggestive of schizophrenia, but whose total duration of illness falls between 1 month and 6 months (option C). Brief psychotic disorder (option D) has a maximum duration of 1 month, and the diagnosis of schizophrenia (option A) is reserved for patients whose total duration of illness exceeds 6 months. Schizoaffective disorder (option B) and bipolar disorder (option E) are not appropriate diagnoses in the absence of mood symptoms. **(pp. 131–133)**

5.12   Which of the following risk factors is associated with poor outcome in schizophrenia?

A. Female sex.
B. Insidious onset of symptoms.
C. Short prodrome.

D. Currently married.

E. Late onset.

The correct response is option B: Insidious onset of symptoms.

Insidious onset of symptoms in schizophrenia is associated with poor outcome (option B). Options A and C–E are all associated with better outcomes. **(Table 5–5 [Features associated with good and poor outcome in schizophrenia], p. 142)**

5.13   Which of the following individuals has the *lowest* risk for developing schizophrenia?

A. Sibling of a person with schizophrenia.

B. Child of parents each having schizophrenia.

C. Identical twin of a person with schizophrenia.

D. Person having a sibling with schizophrenia and one parent with schizophrenia.

E. Child with one parent with schizophrenia.

The correct response is option E: Child with one parent with schizophrenia.

Offspring of parents who each have schizophrenia and identical twins of a person with schizophrenia carry a 46% risk for schizophrenia (options B, C). Siblings of persons with schizophrenia have about a 10% risk for schizophrenia (option A). Persons with one sibling and one parent affected by schizophrenia have a 17% risk for schizophrenia (option D). Children with one parent with schizophrenia have a 5%–6% risk for schizophrenia (option E). **(pp. 144–145)**

5.14   Which of the following vulnerability genes associated with schizophrenia has a known direct effect on dopamine production?

A. Catechol-O-methyltransferase *(COMT)*.

B. Neuregulin 1 *(NRG1)*.

C. D-Amino acid oxidase activator *(DAOA)*.

D. Metabotropic glutamate receptor 3 *(GRM3)*.

E. None of the above.

The correct response is option A: Catechol-O-methyltransferase *(COMT)*.

COMT affects dopamine production (option A). Options B–E have effects on GABA (γ-aminobutyric acid)–ergic and glutamatergic neurotransmission, which are also thought to be dysfunctional in schizophrenia. **(p. 145)**

5.15   Which of the following brain abnormalities in schizophrenia is associated with poor premorbid functioning, negative symptoms, poor response to treatment, and cognitive impairment?

A. Sulcal enlargement.
B. Cerebellar atrophy.
C. Decreased size of frontal lobe.
D. Ventricular enlargement.
E. Decreased size of thalamus.

The correct response is option D: Ventricular enlargement.

Ventricular enlargement in schizophrenia is associated with poor premorbid functioning, negative symptoms, poor response to treatment, and cognitive impairment (option D). Options A–C and E reflect other brain abnormalities that have been associated with schizophrenia but have not been specifically tied to poor outcome or negative symptoms. **(pp. 145–146)**

5.16   Which of the following mechanisms of action has been hypothesized to explain the effectiveness of antipsychotic drugs?

A. Dopamine (D_2) receptor blockade.
B. 5-Hydroxytryptamine (serotonin) type 2 receptor (5-HT_2) blockade.
C. Glutamate receptor blockade.
D. Inhibition of serotonin reuptake.
E. Inhibition of dopamine reuptake.

The correct response is option A: Dopamine (D_2) receptor blockade.

The main mechanism of action of antipsychotic drugs is thought to be their ability to block D_2 receptors (option A). Second-generation antipsychotics also block 5-HT_2 receptors (option B). Glutamate is thought to play a role in schizophrenia, but agents that affect glutamatergic neurotransmission have no current role in the treatment of schizophrenia (option C). SSRI antidepressants inhibit reuptake of serotonin (option D). The antidepressant bupropion is known to block dopamine reuptake (option E). **(pp. 147–148, 559–560)**

5.17 Which of the following psychosocial treatments is known to reduce rates of relapse in schizophrenia?

A. Cognitive-behavioral therapy.
B. Interpersonal psychotherapy.
C. Social skills training.
D. Family therapy.
E. Vocational rehabilitation.

The correct response is option D: Family therapy.

Family therapy, combined with antipsychotic medication, has been shown to reduce relapse rates in schizophrenia (option D). Families need realistic and accurate information about the symptoms, course of illness, and available treatments. They also will benefit from learning how to improve communications with their schizophrenic relative and how to provide constructive support. Although options A–C and E may have value, their effectiveness in reducing relapse rate is not established. **(pp. 149–150)**

5.18 Which of the following features is consistent with a diagnosis of schizoaffective disorder but not major depression or bipolar disorder?

A. Manic episodes accompanied by hallucinations and delusions.
B. Depressive episodes accompanied by hallucinations and delusions.
C. Hallucinations and delusions for at least 2 weeks in the absence of a major mood episode.
D. Presence of a mixed mood episode accompanied by hallucinations and delusions.
E. Symptoms of a major mood episode present for 25% of the total duration of the illness.

The correct response is option C: Hallucinations and delusions for at least 2 weeks in the absence of a major mood episode.

The hallmark of schizoaffective disorder is the presence of either a depressive or a manic episode concurrent with symptoms characteristic of schizophrenia, such as delusions, hallucinations, or disorganized speech. Hallucinations or delusions must be present for 2 weeks or more in the absence of prominent mood symptoms (option C), but mood symptoms must be present for a majority of the total duration of the illness (option E). If the total duration of the mood episodes is less than 50% of the total duration of the illness, schizophrenia is the likely diagnosis. Options A, B, and D are consistent with a diagnosis of a psychotic mood disorder. **(pp. 152–154)**

— CHAPTER 6 —

Mood Disorders

6.1   Who first differentiated bipolar disorder from schizophrenia?

A. Eugen Bleuler.
B. Emil Kraepelin.
C. Sigmund Freud.
D. Kurt Schneider.
E. Carl Jung.

The correct response is option B: Emil Kraepelin.

Kraepelin differentiated bipolar disorder from schizophrenia (option B), although the terms he used at the time were *manic-depressive insanity* and *dementia praecox,* respectively. Bleuler (option A) coined the term *schizophrenia.* Schneider (option D) is noted for identifying "first-rank" symptoms thought to be pathognomonic for schizophrenia. Freud and Jung (options C, E) were famous psychoanalysts who made important contributions to psychiatry but who had no role in separating bipolar disorder from schizophrenia. **(pp. 136, 138 [Chapter 5], 155)**

6.2   Bipolar II disorder first appeared in which edition of the DSM?

A. DSM-I.
B. DSM-II.
C. DSM-III.
D. DSM-IV.
E. DSM-5.

The correct response is option D: DSM-IV.

Bipolar II disorder did not appear until DSM-IV, and it continues to be included in DSM-5. It is important to remember that DSM-I and DSM-II had broader definitions for mood and other disorders, and criteria sets first appeared in 1980 with DSM-III. **(p. 155)**

6.3   What is the minimum duration of a manic episode?

    A. 12 hours.
    B. 1–2 days.
    C. 4 days.
    D. 7 days.
    E. 2 weeks.

The correct response is option D: 7 days.

A manic episode must last at least 7 days according to DSM-5. A hypomanic episode must last for at least 4 days. A major depressive episode must last at least 2 weeks. In the case of mood reactivity lasting from hours up to a day or two, consider affective instability associated with a personality disorder such as borderline personality disorder or cyclothymia. **(pp. 156–157, 161–162)**

6.4   Which of the following features is consistent with a hypomanic episode but *not* a manic episode?

    A. Presence of psychotic symptoms such as hallucinations and delusions.
    B. Duration of at least 1 week.
    C. Elevated mood.
    D. Decreased need for sleep.
    E. Lack of marked social and occupational dysfunction.

The correct response is option E: Lack of marked social and occupational dysfunction.

Hypomanic episodes are different from manic episodes because they do not cause as much social or occupational dysfunction (option E), nor do they typically result in psychiatric hospitalization. Hypomanic episodes are not associated with psychotic symptoms, but psychotic symptoms can occur in manic episodes (option A). Hypomanic episodes must last at least 4 days, but they do not have a specified maximum duration in DSM-5 (option B). Elevated mood and decreased need for sleep (options C, D) can occur in both manic and hypomanic episodes. **(pp. 156–157)**

6.5 A 28-year-old man is brought to the emergency room by the police for a psychiatric evaluation after his neighbors reported that he was behaving erratically. He is irritable and displays pressured speech, and he has only slept a few hours in the past several days. He believes the FBI has implanted a microchip in his brain to record his thoughts and send him messages. He has been spending several hours each day making blueprints for lethal booby traps for his home to protect himself against government agents. He derails frequently in conversation. His physical examination is significant for dental caries, and his urine drug screen is positive for amphetamines. Why would it be premature to diagnose this patient with bipolar I disorder based on this presentation?

A. Presence of psychosis.
B. Persecutory delusions.
C. Mood is irritable rather than elevated.
D. Amphetamines present in drug screen.
E. Lack of grandiosity.

The correct response is option D: Amphetamines present in drug screen.

Without further information, it is premature to diagnose this patient with bipolar disorder, because methamphetamine intoxication can induce manic symptoms (option D). Per DSM-5, it must be determined that manic symptoms are not attributable to the physiological effects of a substance. In this case, collateral information about the time course of illness should be obtained, because patients with bipolar disorder are often disinhibited and more likely to use illicit drugs during manic episodes. Options A, B, C, and E do not rule out bipolar disorder. As a side note, severe paranoia and dental caries are suggestive of a methamphetamine use disorder. **(pp. 156–157)**

6.6 Which of the following features is more characteristic of bipolar II disorder than bipolar I disorder?

A. Multiple hospitalizations.
B. Depressive episodes more prominent during the course of illness.

C. Presence of psychotic symptoms.
D. Lack of a comorbid substance use disorder.
E. Better response to lithium.

The correct response is option B: Depressive episodes more prominent during the course of illness.

Bipolar II disorder may have more prominent depressive episodes in the natural course of illness (option B), although both disorders include major depressive episodes. Bipolar II disorder is often associated with a comorbid substance use disorder (option D). Hospitalizations for mania (option A) and presence of psychotic symptoms (option B) are more characteristic of bipolar I disorder. It has not been established that patients with bipolar II disorder have better response to lithium than patients with bipolar I disorder (option E). **(p. 161)**

6.7   A 10-year-old boy is brought to his family physician by his parents. He has had recurrent severe behavioral outbursts at home and at school several times a week for the past several years. Outbursts are typically in reaction to minor disappointments or when he is asked to do routine chores. His parents did not seek attention for this problem because they thought he would outgrow it. Between outbursts, the boy's mood is "grumpy." What is the most likely diagnosis?

A. Disruptive mood dysregulation disorder.
B. Bipolar II disorder.
C. Major depressive disorder.
D. Persistent depressive disorder.
E. Unspecified depressive disorder.

The correct response is option A: Disruptive mood dysregulation disorder.

Disruptive mood dysregulation disorder is new to DSM-5 for children and adolescents with recurrent severe behavioral outbursts. Prior to DSM-5, many of these children received a diagnosis of bipolar disorder even though they tended not to develop a typical adult bipolar disorder characterized by recurrent manic and depressive episodes. A disruptive mood dysregulation disorder diagnosis can coexist with other depressive disorders, but in this case it is the primary diagnosis, because the information in the vignette is insufficient to diagnose a comorbid depressive disorder. (pp. 162–164)

6.8   A 35-year-old woman comes to your clinic to establish care. She reports that she has been depressed since adolescence with ongoing symptoms of low mood throughout the day, feelings of worthlessness, hypersomnia, low energy, and poor concentration. She does not remember any recent period in the past several years that she was free of depression. What is the best diagnosis?

A. Major depressive disorder.
B. Persistent depressive disorder.
C. Disruptive mood dysregulation disorder.
D. Unspecified depressive disorder.
E. Bipolar II disorder.

The correct response is option B: Persistent depressive disorder.

Patients with continuous symptoms of depression for 2 years or more should be diagnosed with persistent depressive disorder (option B). Only two depressive symptoms are required for the diagnosis, but patients whose symptoms meet full criteria for a major depressive episode should be diagnosed with persistent depressive disorder rather than major depressive disorder (option A) to indicate the chronicity of their illness. Disruptive mood dysregulation disorder (option C) is a diagnosis for children and adolescents with severe, persistent irritability. There is no evidence of hypomania, so bipolar II disorder (option E) is not appropriate. Because this patient meets criteria for persistent depressive disorder, this diagnosis should be used rather than unspecified depressive disorder (option D), which is a diagnosis of exclusion. (pp. 171–173)

6.9   A 30-year-old man comes to your clinic seeking help for depression. He has been feeling depressed most of the day for the past 3 weeks. He complains of restless sleep, low energy, poor concentration, and decreased appetite. He has lost interest in his work, and he spends most of his time watching TV, although with poor attention. He has lost 5 lbs. since this episode started. He has had thoughts of wanting to hang himself, but he does not think he would actually try to kill himself because of his family. This is his fourth episode of depression since adolescence. Prior episodes have resolved spontaneously within a few months, and he is symptom free between episodes. What is the best diagnosis?

A. Disruptive mood dysregulation disorder.
B. Bipolar I disorder.
C. Major depressive disorder.
D. Persistent depressive disorder.
E. Unspecified depressive disorder.

The correct response is option C: Major depressive disorder.

The patient's symptoms meet criteria for major depressive disorder (option C). The patient does not have persistent depressive disorder (option D) because his symptoms are episodic rather than chronic. There is no evidence of a bipolar disorder (option B). Disruptive mood dysregulation disorder (option A) is a diagnosis for highly irritable children, and unspecified depressive disorder (option E) is a diagnosis of exclusion. **(pp. 164–166)**

6.10   A 60-year-old woman develops depressive symptoms following the death of her husband. She has trouble sleeping, feelings of guilt, low energy, decreased appetite, and difficulty paying attention in conversations. She has not had a prior episode of depression, and she is not suicidal. Her symptoms have been ongoing for 3 weeks. What is the best diagnosis?

A. Bereavement.
B. Major depressive disorder.
C. Unspecified depressive disorder.
D. Persistent depressive disorder.
E. Bipolar II disorder.

The correct response is option B: Major depressive disorder.

According to DSM-5, patients who develop symptoms of a major depressive episode due to the loss of a loved one should receive the diagnosis of major depressive disorder (option B) rather than bereavement (option A), which represents a change from DSM-IV. The vignette does not provide evidence of mania or hypomania, and because the patient's symptoms are episodic rather than chronic, persistent depressive disorder is not appropriate (options

D, E). The normal and expected response to an event involving significant loss (e.g., bereavement), including feelings of intense sadness, rumination about the loss, insomnia, poor appetite, and weight loss, may resemble a depressive episode. The presence of symptoms such as feelings of worthlessness, suicidal ideas (as distinct from wanting to join a deceased loved one), psychomotor retardation, and severe impairment of overall function suggest the presence of a major depressive episode in addition to the normal response to a significant loss. Unspecified depressive disorder is inappropriate because it is a diagnosis of exclusion (option C). **(pp. 165–166)**

6.11 What does it mean for a patient with bipolar disorder to have "rapid cycling"?

A. Severe mood swings throughout the day.
B. Switching between mania and depression several times throughout a week.
C. At least four distinct mood episodes (mania, depression, etc.) in 1 year.
D. At least four distinct mood episodes (mania, depression, etc.) in 1 month.
E. None of the above.

The correct response is option C: At least four distinct mood episodes (mania, depression, etc.) in 1 year.

Rapid cycling indicates the presence of at least four distinct mood episodes in 1 year (option C). Rapid-cycling bipolar disorder is a particularly severe form of the disorder and is associated with a younger age at onset, more frequent depressive episodes, and greater risk for suicide attempts than other forms of the disorder. **(p. 177)**

6.12 A major depressive episode characterized by interpersonal rejection sensitivity, increased appetite, and hypersomnia indicates which of the following?

A. Atypical features.
B. Melancholic features.
C. Catatonic features.

D. Diurnal variation.

E. None of the above.

The correct response is option A: Atypical features.

Interpersonal rejection insensitivity, increased appetite, and hypersomnia indicate the presence of atypical features (option A). Melancholic features (option B) are inability to respond to pleasurable stimuli, terminal insomnia, anorexia, excessive guilt, diurnal variation (worse in morning), and marked psychomotor symptoms. Catatonic features (option C) would include somnolence and waxy flexibility. Diurnal variation (option D) is not a specifier for mood episodes. **(pp. 175–176)**

6.13   What is the lifetime prevalence for major depression?

A. 3%.

B. 10%.

C. 17%.

D. 38%.

E. >50%.

The correct response is option C: 17%.

The National Comorbidity Study reported a lifetime prevalence of nearly 17% for major depression. **(p. 179)**

6.14   Which of the following medications is *least* appropriate for the treatment of acute mania?

A. Carbamazepine.

B. Lithium.

C. Second-generation antipsychotic.

D. Gabapentin.

E. Valproate.

The correct response is option D: Gabapentin.

All of the options except for gabapentin have been shown effective for mania. **(p. 184)**

6.15   What class of medication is the first-line treatment for depression?

A. Second-generation antipsychotic.
B. Selective serotonin reuptake inhibitor (SSRI).
C. Tricyclic antidepressant.
D. Serotonin-norepinephrine reuptake inhibitor.
E. Monoamine oxidase inhibitor.

The correct response is option B: Selective serotonin reuptake inhibitor (SSRI).

Treatment should begin with one of the SSRIs because they are well tolerated and safe in overdose (option B). Low dosages are generally effective, and frequent dosage adjustments are usually unnecessary. Although the SSRIs are relatively safe in overdose compared with the older tricyclic antidepressants and monoamine oxidase inhibitors, they have also been reported to increase the risk for impulsive behavior and even suicidality in persons age 24 or younger. Therefore, patients treated with SSRIs should be carefully monitored. The other response options are effective, but their use is limited by their side effect profiles and concerns for safety, thus making them second-line treatment options. **(pp. 184–186)**

— CHAPTER 7 —

Anxiety Disorders

7.1   A 7-year-old girl is brought to a therapist by her parents because
      of she refuses to attend school. She has pretended to be sick
      ("Mommy, my tummy hurts") several times each week for the
      past month to avoid going to school. She reports fear of being
      away from her mother during the day, and she reports nightmares
      of "bad accidents" happening to her mother. What is the most
      likely diagnosis?

      A. Generalized anxiety disorder.
      B. Social anxiety disorder.
      C. Separation anxiety disorder.
      D. Panic disorder.
      E. Specific phobia.

      The correct response is option C: Separation anxiety disorder.

      Patients with separation anxiety disorder show developmentally
      inappropriate anxiety about being apart from an attachment fig-
      ure, and children with this disorder may show school avoidance
      (option C). Patients with generalized anxiety disorder (option A)
      have pervasive anxiety in regard to multiple life areas. Social
      anxiety disorder (option B) is a generalized or circumscribed anx-
      iety with regard to social situations. Patients with panic disorder
      (option D) have brief spells of intense anxiety and autonomic hy-
      perarousal. Patients with a specific phobia (option E) have intense
      anxiety in response to a specific stimulus. In this case, school
      phobia is a symptom of separation anxiety rather than a phobia
      in itself. **(pp. 192–195)**

7.2　A teacher asks the parents of a 10-year-old boy to meet with her. She reports that since the boy started at the school 2 months ago, he has barely said a word and participates minimally in classroom activities. The parents report that, on the contrary, the boy is very talkative at home and they haven't noticed any areas of concern. What is the most likely diagnosis?

A. Generalized anxiety disorder.
B. Social anxiety disorder.
C. Separation anxiety disorder.
D. Selective mutism.
E. Specific phobia.

The correct response is option D: Selective mutism.

Selective mutism is characterized by a persistent failure to speak in a situation in which speaking is expected when speech is normal in certain other environments, such as the home (option D). Patients with separation anxiety disorder (option C) show age-inappropriate anxiety about being apart from an attachment figure, and children with this disorder may show school avoidance. Patients with generalized anxiety disorder (option A) have pervasive anxiety in regard to multiple life areas. Social anxiety disorder (option B) is a generalized or circumscribed anxiety with regard to social situations; however, this patient's failure to speak is more characteristic of selective mutism. Patients with a specific phobia (option E) have intense anxiety in response to a specific stimulus. **(pp. 195–196)**

7.3　What is the primary fear that underlies social anxiety disorder?

A. Social situations.
B. Intimacy.
C. Sexual inadequacy.
D. Public humiliation.
E. Narcissistic injury.

The correct response is option D: Public humiliation.

Social anxiety is based on a fear of public embarrassment (option D); the fear of social situations (option A) is secondary to this. These persons also commonly fear performance situations such as speaking in public, eating in restaurants, writing in front of other persons, or using public restrooms. Sometimes the fear becomes generalized, so that phobic persons avoid most social situations. While intimacy (option B) and feelings of sexual inadequacy (option C) may occur in socially phobic persons, they are not the primary motivating fear. Narcissistic injury (option E) is not associated with social anxiety disorder. **(pp. 197–199)**

7.4   What is the typical age at onset for social anxiety disorder?

A. Preschool years.
B. Elementary school age.
C. Adolescence.
D. Early adulthood.
E. Middle adulthood.

The correct response is option C: Adolescence.

Social anxiety disorder begins during adolescence, and almost always before age 25. Specific phobias often have an onset in childhood. **(p. 199)**

7.5   All but which of the following medication classes is effective in treating social anxiety disorder?

A. Selective serotonin reuptake inhibitors (SSRIs).
B. Monoamine oxidase inhibitors (MAOIs).
C. Tricyclic antidepressants (TCAs).
D. β-Blockers.
E. Benzodiazepines.

The correct response is option C: Tricyclic antidepressants.

Several of the SSRIs have a U.S. Food and Drug Administration (FDA) indication to treat social anxiety disorder (option A). The MAOIs and benzodiazepines (options B, E) are likely effective but are second-line choices. TCAs are probably less effective (option C), and socially anxious patients may be overly sensitive to their activating side effects (e.g., jitteriness). β-Blocking drugs (option D) are effective for the short-term treatment of performance-related anxiety but are otherwise ineffective for social anxiety disorder. **(pp. 201–202)**

7.6   A 24-year-old woman presents to the emergency room complaining of the sudden onset of shortness of breath, dizziness, diaphoresis, chest pain, and a sense of impending doom. Her medical work-up is negative, and her symptoms resolve within 30 minutes. She has had multiple prior episodes and fears her next spell. She avoids public places for fear of having an episode in public. What is the most likely diagnosis?

A. Generalized anxiety disorder.
B. Specific phobia.
C. Panic disorder.
D. Separation anxiety disorder.
E. Social anxiety disorder.

The correct response is option C: Panic disorder.

This patient is presenting with classic symptoms of panic disorder (option C), as well as reporting multiple prior panic attacks and preoccupation with having subsequent attacks. Panic attacks typically reach their peak in 10 minutes. Agoraphobia has developed secondary to the panic attacks, so specific phobia (option B) is not the primary diagnosis. Patients with separation anxiety disorder (option D) show age-inappropriate anxiety about being apart from an attachment figure, and children with this disorder may show school avoidance. Patients with generalized anxiety disorder (option A) have pervasive anxiety in regard to multiple life areas. Social anxiety disorder (option E) is a generalized or circumscribed anxiety with regard to social situations. **(pp. 202–205)**

7.7   Which of the following medications is the best long-term treatment for specific phobia?

A. Fluoxetine.
B. Lorazepam.
C. Sertraline.
D. Alprazolam.
E. None of the above.

The correct response is option E: None of the above.

Benzodiazepines provide short-term relief from a specific phobia, and long-term use is not recommended because of habituation and abuse potential. Otherwise, medications are not generally effective treatments for specific phobia. Patients can benefit from behavioral therapies. **(p. 202)**

7.8   Which two psychiatric disorders are the most likely to be comorbid with panic disorder?

A. Generalized anxiety disorder and major depressive disorder.
B. Generalized anxiety disorder and social anxiety disorder.
C. Major depressive disorder and alcohol use disorder.
D. Specific phobia and alcohol use disorder.
E. Persistent depressive disorder and generalized anxiety disorder.

The correct response is option C: Major depressive disorder and alcohol use disorder.

The most common comorbid psychiatric disorders are major depression and alcohol use disorders. Major depression occurs in up to half of the patients with panic disorder and may be severe. Misuse of alcohol or other drugs complicates panic disorder in about 20% of the cases and may start in an attempt at self-medication. This complication is important to keep in mind when evaluating patients who abuse substances, because they may also have an underlying, treatable anxiety disorder. A person with panic disorder may also have another anxiety disorder requiring evaluation and treatment, such as social anxiety disorder or generalized anxiety disorder. **(pp. 206–207)**

7.9   What substance has been implicated in the "false suffocation alarm" theory of panic disorder?

A. CO_2.
B. O_2.
C. Sodium lactate.
D. Melatonin.
E. CO.

The correct response is option A: CO_2.

Although the etiology of panic disorder is unknown, the observation that exposure to 5% CO_2 induces panic attacks has led to the "false suffocation alarm" theory. The theory posits that patients with panic disorder are hypersensitive to CO_2 because they have an overly sensitive brain stem suffocation alarm system that produces respiratory distress, hyperventilation, and anxiety. **(p. 208)**

7.10   A 20-year-old college student develops symptoms of intense anxiety, racing heart, dizziness, diaphoresis, and shortness of breath. The symptoms resolve within less than 30 minutes. Prior to developing these symptoms, he had consumed several cups of coffee in an effort to stay up late studying for an exam. He had not had prior episodes. What is the most likely diagnosis?

A. Panic disorder.
B. Specific phobia.
C. Social phobia.
D. Substance-induced anxiety disorder.
E. Generalized anxiety disorder.

The correct response is option D: Substance-induced anxiety disorder.

This patient has a caffeine-induced anxiety disorder because his panic attack is attributable to the physiological effects of caffeine rather than a primary panic disorder (option C). The patient does not exhibit symptoms of the other anxiety disorders in options A, B, D, and E. **(p. 210)**

7.11   What is the literal meaning of the term *agoraphobia*?

A. Fear of people.
B. Fear of crowds.
C. Fear of open spaces.
D. Fear of the marketplace.
E. Fear of enclosed spaces.

The correct response is option D: Fear of the marketplace.

Agoraphobia's Greek roots mean "fear of the marketplace." **(p. 211)**

7.12   A 30-year-old woman complains to her new family physician of feeling "wound up" all the time. She describes herself as a "worrier" and feels she has always been this way, always worrying about "everything." She has chronic insomnia and reports having muscle tension in her neck and shoulders. She has a hard time concentrating. She drinks a cup of coffee in the morning but otherwise does not use stimulants. She denies depression or substance abuse. What is the most likely diagnosis?

A. Separation anxiety disorder.
B. Generalized anxiety disorder.
C. Substance-induced anxiety disorder.
D. Agoraphobia.
E. Panic disorder.

The correct response is option B: Generalized anxiety disorder.

Patients with generalized anxiety disorder have a chronic tendency to worry and to feel on edge much of the time; they may have trouble concentrating, muscle tension, and/or insomnia (option B). Separation anxiety (option A) is the tendency to have intense anxiety about separation from an object of attachment. The patient in this scenario does not drink enough caffeine to account for substance-induced anxiety disorder (option C). Agoraphobia (option D) is fear of being in public places, and some patients find it very difficult to leave home. Panic disorder (option E) involves having recurrent panic attacks and a secondary fear of having subsequent attacks. **(pp. 212–215)**

7.13   The treatment of generalized anxiety disorder usually involves individual psychotherapy in addition to which of the following medications?

A. Buspirone.
B. Escitalopram.
C. Venlafaxine.
D. Duloxetine.
E. All of the above.

The correct response is option E: All of the above.

The treatment of generalized anxiety disorder usually involves individual psychotherapy and medication. All medications listed have been FDA approved to treat the disorder (option E). Patients should be educated about the chronic nature of the disorder and the tendency of symptoms to wax and wane, often along with external stressors that the patient may be experiencing. Behavior therapy may help the patient to recognize and control anxiety symptoms. Relaxation training, re-breathing exercises, and meditation can be easily taught and may be effective, especially if the condition is mild. Benzodiazepine tranquillizers should be avoided because of their tendency to induce tolerance and dependence. Their use in these patients should be limited. **(pp. 215–216)**

— CHAPTER 8 —

Obsessive-Compulsive and Related Disorders

8.1   Which of the following is *not* considered an obsession according to DSM-5?

A. Recurrent concerns about germs or contamination.
B. Fixation on the appearance of a particular body part.
C. Intrusive and disturbing thoughts about a loved one being murdered.
D. Obsessive desire to achieve an ambitious career goal to fulfill long-standing dreams.
E. Need to collect worthless items and being unable to throw things away.

The correct response is option D: Obsessive desire to achieve an ambitious career goal to fulfill long-standing dreams.

Obsessions are recurrent and persistent ideas, thoughts, impulses, or images that are experienced as intrusive and inappropriate and that cause marked anxiety or distress. This is in contrast to layman's usage of the term *obsession*. Option D is not an obsession because it is not experienced as intrusive and inappropriate. Options A, B, C, and E are consistent with major categories of obsessions: contamination, somatic, aggression, and hoarding, respectively. **(pp. 220–222)**

8.2 Which of the following is *not* a common compulsive ritual?

    A. Handwashing.
    B. Counting.
    C. Gambling.
    D. Checking.
    E. Symmetrical arranging.

The correct response is option C: Gambling.

Options A, B, D, and E are common compulsions. Compulsions are repetitive and intentional behaviors (or mental acts) performed in response to obsessions or according to certain rules that must be applied rigidly. Compulsions are meant to neutralize or reduce discomfort or to prevent a dreaded event or situation. The rituals are not connected in a realistic way to the event or situation or are clearly excessive. None of these descriptors apply to gambling, which is voluntary and perceived as pleasurable (option C). **(pp. 222–223)**

8.3 A 34-year-old man with generalized anxiety disorder tells his psychiatrist he is worried that he may have obsessive-compulsive disorder (OCD) after reading an article on the Internet. He checks his door locks repetitively each morning before leaving for work, which may take 5–10 minutes. He worries that burglars could enter the house, but he is able to put the thought out of his mind after leaving his home. He has had these behaviors since adolescence. There is no family history of OCD. On the basis of this information, what should the psychiatrist tell this patient?

    A. We should start clomipramine for OCD.
    B. OCD is not likely, based on the age at onset of your symptoms.
    C. OCD is not likely, based on your negative family history.
    D. OCD is not likely because your symptoms are so mild.
    E. OCD is not likely, based on your established diagnosis of generalized anxiety disorder.

The correct response is option D: OCD is not likely because your symptoms are so mild.

This patient should not be diagnosed with OCD because his symptoms are mild and do not cause significant impairment (option

D). Many psychiatrically healthy individuals have simple rituals such as checking locks. Compulsive behaviors should occupy a significant amount of time (1 hour a day or more) for a diagnosis of OCD. Age at onset and family history (options B, C) are not listed as part of the diagnostic criteria. The patient's symptoms may be considered subclinical because, although they are not explained by his diagnosis of generalized anxiety disorder (option E), they are not impairing. Finally, clomipramine, while an effective medication for OCD, is not used in subclinical cases (option A). **(pp. 220–224)**

8.4   A 25-year-old man sees a psychiatrist for help for his OCD. He spends over 2–3 hours each day arranging his bookshelves at home and is fed up with his need to do this. He feels he is unable to stop his behavior and is afraid to have people over to his home for fear they might "mess up" the shelves. He has never sought treatment because he thought he could handle it on his own. Which of the following options is a reasonable treatment strategy for this patient?

A. Clomipramine.
B. Fluoxetine.
C. Behavior therapy.
D. Clomipramine and behavior therapy.
E. All of the above.

The correct response is option E: All of the above.

The treatment of OCD usually involves medication and behavior therapy (option E). Selective serotonin reuptake inhibitors (SSRIs) such as fluoxetine are particularly effective and several are FDA approved for the treatment of OCD. Clomipramine, a tricyclic antidepressant that is a relatively specific serotonin reuptake blocker, is also FDA approved to treat OCD. However, because of its many side effects, it is used less frequently than are the SSRIs. Typically, higher dosages of the SSRIs are needed to treat OCD than to treat major depression, and response is often delayed. With behavior therapy, which consists of exposure and response prevention, a patient might be exposed to a dreaded situation, event, or stimulus by various techniques (e.g., imaginal exposure, systematic desensitization, flooding) and then prevented from carrying out the compulsive behavior that usually results. Treatment results are fairly comparable for medication and behavior therapy, and the combination is probably most effective. **(pp. 227–228)**

8.5   A patient comes to establish care with a new psychiatrist for treatment of OCD. He has been to several psychiatrists and therapists in the past 10 years, but he is frustrated because none of the treatments has been curative. How should the psychiatrist respond to this patient's concern?

A. Review the patient's adherence to specific medications.
B. Ask how long the patient has been able to stay in exposure therapy.
C. Recommend a new medication.
D. Inform the patient that OCD tends to be chronic.
E. None of the above.

The correct response is option D: Inform the patient that OCD tends to be chronic.

OCD is chronic in nearly all cases; therefore, patients should not expect treatments to be curative (option D). Once it has been established that the goal of treatment is to reduce symptoms and improve quality of life rather than provide a cure, options A–C all become reasonable. **(pp. 224–228)**

8.6   Which of the following disorders appears to be genetically linked with OCD?

A. Pediatric autoimmune neuropsychiatric disorders associated with streptococcal infections (PANDAS).
B. Tourette's disorder.
C. Epilepsy.
D. Huntington's disease.
E. Sydenham's chorea.

The correct response is option B: Tourette's disorder.

OCD has a considerable genetic component as characterized by family and twin studies, and appears linked with Tourette's disorder (option B). PANDAS (option A) is an acquired form of OCD that occurs in children following group A β-streptococcal infection. Epilepsy, Huntington's disease, and Sydenham's chorea have been associated with OCD, but there is no evidence for a genetic link (options C, D, E). **(pp. 225–226)**

8.7   A 17-year-old woman is brought to a psychiatrist because of the concerns of her parents. She spends an inordinate amount of time staring at her nose in the mirror and has been saving income from a part-time job for a rhinoplasty. The patient says her nose is ugly and that her classmates stare at it, making fun of her through coded references. She cannot be reassured by her family that her nose looks normal and is even attractive. On examination, the nose appears unremarkable. She reports feeling demoralized by her concerns about her nose but has no history of depression, and she is not psychotic. There is no evidence of a thought disorder or disorganization. What is the best diagnosis?

A. OCD with somatic obsessions.
B. Obsessive-compulsive personality disorder.
C. Delusional disorder, somatic type.
D. Body dysmorphic disorder.
E. Schizophrenia.

The correct response is option D: Body dysmorphic disorder.

Patients with body dysmorphic disorder are preoccupied with an imagined defect or flaw in physical appearance (option D). Because of this belief, body dysmorphic disorder should be the primary diagnosis in this case and not delusional disorder, somatic type (option C). Because of the circumscribed nature of her symptoms, body dysmorphic disorder is a better diagnosis than OCD with somatic obsessions (option A). Patients with obsessive-compulsive personality disorder have a rigid, perfectionistic pattern of behavior (option B), but this usually has nothing to do with body concerns. Apart from her somatic preoccupation, this patient does not have symptoms to suggest schizophrenia such as hallucinations, disorganization, or a formal thought disorder (option E). **(pp. 228–231)**

8.8   A 30-year-old man sees a psychiatrist at his wife's insistence. She is concerned about the possibility of him having OCD after watching a TV program about hoarding. He has an extensive video game collection that he has been accumulating since age 7. His collection is neatly arranged on shelves that do not take up much space. He is proud of his collection, and he would never think about getting rid of a single title because he sees no reason to do so. He enjoys playing video games for an hour or so each day, but otherwise keeps busy with work. He is tight with money and insists on doing many household chores himself because he believes his family can't ever do things to his standards. He has rigid political ideas that he is happy to share with others on his favorite social networking site. He does not feel that he has a significant problem with depression or anxiety. What is the most likely diagnosis?

A. OCD.
B. Obsessive-compulsive personality disorder.
C. Hoarding disorder.
D. Gaming addiction.
E. Partner relational problem.

The correct response is option B: Obsessive-compulsive personality disorder.

This patient's attitude toward his collecting behavior is not consistent with hoarding disorder, which requires that hoarding result in clutter that compromises the active use of living area (option C). His rigid, perfectionistic personality is consistent with obsessive-compulsive personality disorder (option B), which is an important part of the differential diagnosis of OCD (option A) and related disorders. Because the patient is not bothered by his symptoms and finds enjoyment in his collecting, OCD is not a reasonable choice (option A). The other two response options are not reasonable choices. DSM-5 does not include gaming addiction as an independent disorder, nor does the vignette imply that his use is excessive (option D). The patient and his wife may have marital difficulties that center around the collection, but it does not explain his behavior (option E). **(pp. 227, 231–232)**

8.9   What kind of psychotherapy is recommended for trichotillomania?

A. Supportive psychotherapy.
B. Behavioral therapy.
C. Psychodynamic psychotherapy.
D. Interpersonal psychotherapy.
E. Acceptance and commitment therapy.

The correct response is option B: Behavioral therapy.

Treatment of trichotillomania, or hair-pulling disorder, consists of medication combined with behavioral therapy. With behavior therapy, patients learn to identify when their hair pulling occurs (it is often automatic) and to substitute benign behaviors such as squeezing a ball. Some patients benefit from learning to apply barriers to prevent hair pulling, such as wearing gloves or a hat. These techniques are often referred to as *habit reversal*, and research studies show they can be effective. All the other psychotherapies listed (options A, C, D, E) may be helpful but have not been shown to be effective in treating trichotillomania. **(p. 235)**

8.10 Which tricyclic antidepressant has shown benefit for trichotillo-mania?

A. Imipramine.
B. Doxepin.
C. Clomipramine.
D. Amitriptyline.
E. Nortriptyline.

The correct response is option C: Clomipramine.

Clomipramine has been shown to have benefit for trichotillomania as well as OCD. It works preferentially on the serotonin system. **(p. 235)**

8.11 A 31-year old woman has many open and bleeding sores on her forearms. She has sought help from dermatologists, who have pre-scribed various creams, all to no avail. The last dermatologist in-sisted that the woman seek a psychiatric evaluation. What is the most likely diagnosis?

A. Trichotillomania.
B. Unspecified obsessive-compulsive and related disorder.
C. Excoriation disorder.
D. Delusional disorder, somatic type.
E. OCD.

The correct response is option C: Excoriation disorder.

Excoriation disorder is new to DSM-5. People with this disorder repetitively and compulsively pick at their skin, which leads to tissue damage. There are significant clinical similarities between excoriation disorder and trichotillomania (option A; compulsive hair pulling), and the criteria for the two disorders are similar. In rare cases, stimulants can cause skin-picking behaviors; therefore, stimulant use or abuse needs to be ruled out. Dermatological conditions such as scabies, atopic dermatitis, psoriasis, and blistering skin disorders also need ruling out. Excoriation disorder patients are not delusional (option D), and they do not pick in response to worrisome thoughts (option E). Option B is not reasonable because it is a diagnosis of exclusion. **(pp. 235–236)**

8.12   In excoriation disorder, where is the most common site for skin picking?

A. Face.
B. Hands.
C. Feet.
D. Arms.
E. Torso.

The correct response is option A: Face.

The face is the most commonly site of picking (option A). Other areas such as the hands, fingers, torso, arms, and legs are also common targets. People with this disorder use their fingernails, knives, and even tweezers and pins for picking. Picking may result in significant tissue damage and may lead to medical complications such as localized infections or septicemia. **(p. 236)**

— CHAPTER 9 —

Trauma- and Stressor-Related Disorders

9.1   A 7-year-old boy is brought to a child psychiatrist by his new fos-
      ter parents. He had been removed from his biological parents at
      an early age because of neglect, and he has been in several foster
      homes. They report that he is sullen much of the time and almost
      never smiles. He often becomes irritable, and they are unable to
      console him. He appears to interact normally with his peers. What
      is the most likely diagnosis?

      A. Posttraumatic stress disorder (PTSD).
      B. Autism spectrum disorder.
      C. Reactive attachment disorder.
      D. Adjustment disorder with depressed mood.
      E. Disinhibited social engagement disorder.

      The correct response is option C: Reactive attachment disorder.

      Reactive attachment disorder can develop in children exposed to
      severe negligence. These children do not seek caregiver attention
      as would their peers, nor do they respond to caregiver attempts to
      comfort them. Disinhibited social engagement disorder (option E)
      occurs when a neglected child behaves toward adults in an overly
      familiar fashion. PTSD (option A) involves hypervigilance, avoid-
      ance, and reexperiencing symptoms that develop in response to
      a trauma. Autism spectrum disorder (option B) is an important part
      of the differential of reactive attachment disorder, but the cardinal
      symptoms (social communication, repetitive patterns of behavior)

are not present. Adjustment disorder with depressed mood (option D) is when someone develops limited depressive symptoms in reaction to a stressful event. Given this child's background and presenting symptoms, a diagnosis of reactive attachment better fits the picture than an adjustment disorder (option C). **(pp. 240–244, 255–256)**

9.2   A 6-year-old girl is brought to a child psychiatrist by her new foster parents. She had been removed from her biological parents at an early age because of neglect, and she has been in multiple prior foster homes. Since moving to her new home, her foster parents have noticed that she will initiate conversations with strangers at the supermarket, and she once attempted to go home with another family. During the interview, the child jumps on the psychiatrist's lap and begins stroking her back. Testing has shown that she has a mild intellectual disability, and there is no history of a mood disturbance. What is the best diagnosis?

A. PTSD.
B. Intellectual developmental disorder.
C. Bipolar I disorder.
D. Adjustment disorder with depressed mood.
E. Disinhibited social engagement disorder.

The correct response is option E: Disinhibited social engagement disorder.

Disinhibited social engagement disorder occurs when a neglected child behaves toward adults in an overly familiar fashion (option E). PTSD (option A) involves hypervigilance, avoidance, and re-experiencing symptoms that develop in response to a trauma. Adjustment disorder with depressed mood (option D) is when someone develops limited depressive symptoms in reaction to a stressful event. There is no evidence of a bipolar disorder (option C), although bipolar patients may be disinhibited when manic or hypomanic. The patient has a mild intellectual disability, but this would not explain her behavior (option B). **(pp. 240–244, 255–256)**

9.3   What is the most common precipitating event for women diagnosed with PTSD?

A. Natural disaster.
B. Experiencing a fire.

C. Sexual assault.

D. Hospitalization in an intensive care unit.

E. Combat.

The correct response is option C: Sexual assault.

Physical or sexual assault is the most common precipitating event for women diagnosed with PTSD (option C), although options A, B, D, and E can certainly be sufficient to precipitate the disorder. **(p. 249)**

9.4 Which of the following symptom areas is *not* a required part of the PTSD diagnosis?

A. Reexperiencing of the trauma through intrusive thoughts or dreams.

B. Dissociative symptoms such as derealization or depersonalization.

C. Avoidance of stimuli associated with the event.

D. Negative alterations in mood such as feeling numb or detached from others.

E. Alterations in arousal and reactivity such as irritability/angry outbursts and exaggerated startle response.

The correct response is option B: Dissociative symptoms such as derealization or depersonalization.

Derealization and depersonalization are not required for the PTSD diagnosis (option B), although some patients will have them, and DSM-5 includes a specifier ("with dissociative symptoms") for these patients. Symptoms in options A, C, D, and E are required for the diagnosis of PTSD. **(pp. 245–249)**

9.5 What is the best medication choice for PTSD?

A. Sertraline.

B. Venlafaxine.

C. Diazepam.

D. Prazosin.

E. Lithium.

The correct response is option A: Sertraline.

Selective serotonin reuptake inhibitors (SSRIs), for example, sertraline, are the first-line treatment for PTSD (option A). Venlafaxine (option B) may be effective but is not as well studied. Prazosin (option D) may be helpful for PTSD-related nightmares but is not an established treatment for other symptoms. Lithium (option E) has no role in the treatment of PTSD. Benzodiazepine tranquillizers such as diazepam (option C) may be helpful but should only be used for short-term management of accompanying anxiety because of their potential for habituation and abuse. **(pp. 251–252)**

9.6 A 30-year-old veteran is seen in follow-up for his PTSD precipitated by wartime combat. He reports ongoing disturbing nightmares about his past experiences. He continues to have other symptoms as well, but they are less distressing to him. Which of the following medications is most appropriate to target his chief complaint?

A. Sertraline.
B. Venlafaxine.
C. Clonazepam.
D. Prazosin.
E. Lithium.

The correct response is option D: Prazosin.

Prazosin is an α_1-adrenergic antagonist shown to reduce nightmares associated with PTSD (option D). SSRIs (such as sertraline [option A]) or venlafaxine (option B) are useful medications but have no specific effect on nightmares. Lithium (option E) has no role in the treatment of PTSD. Benzodiazepine tranquillizers such as clonazepam may help reduce anxiety associated with PTSD but have no role in treating accompanying nightmares (option C). **(pp. 251–252)**

9.7 A 24-year-old man seeks help of a psychiatrist because of problems with irritability and feeling "on guard" since a motor vehicle accident 2 weeks earlier. Luckily, he only sustained minor injuries, but his vehicle was destroyed. Since the accident, he has felt out of sorts and has had intrusive memories and nightmares about the event. He has been using public transportation to get to work and now avoids going by the scene of the accident. What is the most likely diagnosis?

A. PTSD.

B. Acute stress disorder.

C. Adjustment disorder with anxious features.

D. Unspecified anxiety disorder.

E. None of the above.

The correct response is option B: Acute stress disorder.

The key difference between acute stress disorder and PTSD is duration of symptoms. PTSD (option A) can only be diagnosed if the symptoms have been ongoing for more than 1 month. Hypervigilance, avoidance, and reexperiencing that occur for the first month following a traumatic experience should be diagnosed as acute stress disorder (option B). The major difference between these diagnoses and adjustment disorder is that with adjustment disorder (option C), the patient develops depressive or anxious symptoms in reaction to a non-life-threatening event, such as a relationship break up. Option D is not appropriate because it is a diagnosis of exclusion. **(p. 254)**

9.8   A 17-year-old boy whose parents divorced 2 months earlier is brought to a therapist by his mother. He has always been a good student, but his grades have dropped, and he has been getting into fights at school over the past month. There is no history of behavioral problems. He says that he isn't depressed, and there have been no changes in his appetite, sleep, or activity level. He answers "I don't know," to most of the therapist's questions. What is the most likely diagnosis?

A. PTSD.

B. Acute stress disorder.

C. Adjustment disorder.

D. Major depression.

E. Reactive attachment disorder.

The correct response is option C: Adjustment disorder.

Acute behavioral changes following an identifiable stressor are suggestive of an adjustment disorder (option C). Adolescents with adjustment disorder are more likely to act out, whereas adults are more likely to develop depression and anxiety. This patient has not experienced a life-threatening event, so PTSD and acute stress disorder (options A, B) are not likely diagnoses. The patient reports that he is not depressed, and there are no vegetative symptoms of depression, so unless the depression is "masked" it is not a reasonable diagnostic choice (option D). Reactive attachment disorder is a diagnosis for children who experience severe neglect who do not show normal attention seeking behavior directed toward their caregivers, so option E is not plausible. **(pp. 252, 255–260)**

9.9 What is the most common stressor for adults with an adjustment disorder?

A. Divorce or separation.
B. Marital problems.
C. Work problems.
D. Financial problems.
E. Moving.

The correct response is option B: Marital problems.

Marital problems are the most frequent cause of adjustment disorders in adults (option B), although options A, C, D, and E are also common stressors. **(Table 9–2 [Stressors occurring in adolescents and adults with adjustment disorders], p. 258)**

9.10 What is the most common stressor to precipitate an adjustment disorder in adolescents?

A. Marital problems in parents.
B. School problems.
C. Drug or alcohol problem.
D. Parental rejection.
E. Boyfriend/girlfriend problems.

The correct response is option B: School problems.

School problems accounted for 60% of adjustment disorders in adolescents (option B), although options A, C, D, and E are common precipitants. **(Table 9–2 [Stressors occurring in adolescents and adults with adjustment disorders], p. 258)**

9.11   Which of the following is required for a diagnosis of adjustment
        disorder?

    A. Identifiable stressor.
    B. Depressive symptoms.
    C. Anxious symptoms.
    D. Disturbance of conduct.
    E. None of the above.

The correct response is option A: Identifiable stressor.

Without an identifiable stressor, there is no adjustment disorder
(option A). The pertinent question for the clinician is, "What is
the patient having trouble adjusting to?" Adjustment disorders
are common particularly in hospital settings. They can manifest
in many ways such as with a disturbance of mood or anxiety or
a conduct disturbance (options B, C, D). **(pp. 255–258)**

9.12   What is the best treatment for an adjustment disorder?

    A. Sedative-hypnotics.
    B. SSRIs.
    C. Antipsychotics.
    D. Supportive therapy.
    E. Cognitive-behavioral therapy.

The correct response is option D: Supportive therapy.

Adjustment disorders should resolve within 6 months of termination of the stressor; therefore, time and supportive therapy are
treatment mainstays (option D). A sedative-hypnotic (option A)
may be helpful if the patient has insomnia as part of the adjustment disorder, but it is not a standard treatment for adjustment
disorder. Antipsychotics (option C) have no role in the treatment
of adjustment disorders. Both SSRIs and cognitive-behavioral
therapy (options B, E) may be useful but are probably not necessary because most adjustment disorders are short-lived and tend
to remit. **(pp. 255, 260)**

CHAPTER 10

Somatic Symptom Disorders and Dissociative Disorders

10.1 A 30-year-old man presents to his primary care physician with a new concern that he may have a brain tumor. He reports that for the past week he has had tingling on his scalp. He had a mild headache the day before that resolved with ibuprofen. At his last visit a few months ago, he was concerned that he had pancreatic cancer because he noticed a small area of yellow discoloration on his upper arm. What is the most likely diagnosis?

A. Somatic symptom disorder.
B. Illness anxiety disorder.
C. Factitious disorder.
D. Conversion disorder.
E. Malingering.

The correct response is option B: Illness anxiety disorder.

Note that most vignettes in this chapter take place in a primary care setting because primary care physicians are more likely to see patients with somatic symptom disorder than are psychiatrists. Patients with these conditions tend not to view them as being psychologically motivated and so rarely seek mental health care for the conditions.

Patients with illness anxiety disorder have recurrent concerns that they may have a serious illness based on mild or absent somatic symptoms (option B). Many of these patients would have received a diagnosis of hypochondriasis in DSM-IV. Patients with somatic symptom disorder (option A) are preoccupied with their somatic symptoms themselves rather than the possibility that they may signify a significant illness. Patients with factitious disorder (option C) feign illness in order to play the patient role. Patients who malinger (option E) feign illness for personal gain. (Malingering is not considered a mental disorder but rather is categorized as a "V/Z code" diagnosis in DSM-5.) Conversion disorder (option D) is a reported disturbance of motor or sensory function that is inconsistent with neurological disease. **(pp. 264, 268–269, 271, 277, 280)**

10.2 A 24-year-old woman is referred to neurology for evaluation of spells that began 2 months earlier. She reports having seizures two or three times a week that are characterized by bilateral arm flapping without impairment of consciousness or loss of bowel or bladder control. The electroencephalogram is negative for epileptiform activity, and routine laboratory studies are unremarkable. What is the most likely diagnosis?

A. Somatic symptom disorder.
B. Convulsive disorder.
C. Factitious disorder.
D. Conversion disorder.
E. Malingering.

The correct response is option D: Conversion disorder.

The patient best fits the diagnosis of conversion disorder, which is a reported disturbance of motor or sensory function that is inconsistent with neurological disease (option D). Her symptoms are widely considered "pseudoseizures," but they are better referred to as "nonepileptic spells" and are not compatible with a true convulsive disorder (option B). They resemble seizures but are unaccompanied by abnormal brain waves. Pseudoseizures often occur in patients with true seizure disorders. Somatic symptom disorder (option A) is defined by the presence of one or more distressing or disruptive somatic symptoms, but the patient's symptoms are better explained as a conversion disorder. The vignette does not suggest symptom falsification, as in factitious disorder (option C), or intentional production of symptoms, as in malingering (option E). **(pp. 271–272)**

10.3   How many somatic symptoms are required to make a DSM-5 diagnosis of somatic symptom disorder?

A. One.
B. Two.
C. Four.
D. Six.
E. Eight.

The correct response is option A: One.

The DSM-5 diagnosis of somatic symptom disorder only requires the presence of a single somatic symptom, which represents a simplification of the more cumbersome DSM-IV construct of somatization disorder. **(p. 264)**

10.4   A 60-year-old man on disability sees his family physician in follow-up for chronic pain. He reports pain in multiple joints, and he frequently requests more opioid pain medications to help with his symptoms. Diagnostic studies show only changes consistent with normal aging. The patient's primary concern is with pain, and there is no evidence that he misuses his medications. He has been amenable to trying interventions such as physical therapy, although they have not produced adequate results. What is the most likely diagnosis?

A. Pain disorder.
B. Somatic symptom disorder.
C. Opioid use disorder.
D. Conversion disorder.
E. Malingering.

The correct response is option B: Somatic symptom disorder.

Patients who would have been diagnosed with pain disorder in DSM-IV now receive the more general diagnosis of somatic symptom disorder (option B). This new diagnosis consolidates DSM-IV's somatization disorder, hypochondriasis, pain disorder (option A), and undifferentiated somatoform disorder. These diagnoses were rarely used and created confusion for clinicians and patients. The new diagnosis is more user-friendly to clinicians and is likely felt to be less stigmatizing to patients. In the vignette, although the patient requests pain medication, there is insufficient information to suggest that he has an opioid use disorder (option C) or that he is feigning symptoms, as in malingering (option E). Conversion disorder (option D) involves symptoms that suggest a neurological condition, such as weakness or paralysis. (pp. 264–266, 271, 280)

10.5   A 19-year-old man presents to his family physician, convinced that his intestines are rotting and that he may already be dead. He is not able to cite any symptoms that give rise to this conviction. Physical examination and routine laboratory tests are normal. The patient does not accept his physician's reassurance that he is healthy. What is the most likely diagnosis?

A. Somatic symptom disorder.
B. Illness anxiety disorder.
C. Schizophrenia.
D. Malingering.
E. Unspecified somatic symptom disorder.

The correct response is option C: Schizophrenia.

The patient is clearly psychotic and has nihilistic delusions. A patient with illness anxiety disorder (option B) is preoccupied with having an illness but is not delusional. A patient with somatic symptom disorder (options A, E) would be preoccupied with one or more symptoms rather than a conviction. Because there is no reason to believe the patient is feigning illness, we can rule out malingering (option D). **(pp. 264, 268, 280)**

10.6   A psychiatrist is asked to consult on a 25-year-old man admitted to a general neurological service for sudden onset of lower-extremity weakness. The patient has reported that he cannot walk, although diagnostic studies have not shown any physical reason to account for the symptoms. The patient asks if he will ever get any better. How should the psychiatrist respond?

A. "Your condition will most likely improve with time."
B. "You will most likely have permanent disability."

C. "Your prognosis is guarded."

D. "It is too early to draw any conclusion."

E. "It will depend on your willingness to engage in cognitive-behavioral therapy."

The correct response is option A: "Your condition will most likely improve with time."

Conversion symptoms are very common in hospitals, and follow-up studies show that most tend to improve or remit spontaneously. Onset may occur at any point throughout life, and although most conversion symptoms are transient, for persons receiving a diagnosis of conversion disorder a favorable outcome is generally associated with acute onset, a precipitating stressor, good premorbid adjustment, and the absence of medical or neurological comorbidity. There are no established treatments for the disorder. **(pp. 271–275)**

10.7   A 55-year-old woman sees her family physician for an annual physical examination. During the review of symptoms, she reports chronic dyspepsia. She had the same complaint during her last three visits. She has not had any visits or phone calls between visits. A medical workup for this complaint was negative 3 years ago. She is not preoccupied with this symptom, and her social and occupational functioning is normal. The physician considers diagnosing somatic symptom disorder because there is no obvious medical explanation for her complaint. Her medical student, fresh from her psychiatry clerkship, objects and says that it would inappropriate. Why so?

A. Patients with somatic symptom disorder must have multiple somatic complaints.

B. The patient's lack of interest in her symptoms makes a conversion disorder more likely.

C. The physician has not investigated possible motivations for secondary gain or to play the patient role.

D. The diagnosis of somatic symptom disorder requires the patient have significant preoccupation or personal investment in his or her symptoms.

E. The medical student is wrong, and it is appropriate to diagnose this patient with somatic symptom disorder.

The correct response is option D: The diagnosis of somatic symptom disorder requires the patient have significant preoccupation or personal investment in his or her symptoms.

A key difference between DSM-5's somatic symptom disorder and the DSM-IV somatoform disorder diagnoses is that now the patient must have excessive thoughts, feelings, or behaviors related to the symptom or symptoms (option E). The woman in the vignette is clearly not preoccupied by the symptom (option D). Further, there is no longer any reliance, as in DSM-IV, on the symptoms being medically unexplained. Only one symptom is required for a diagnosis of somatic symptom disorder (option A), and conversion disorder requires a pseudoneurological symptom (option B), so these diagnoses are not appropriate. There is no evidence that the woman is feigning her symptoms or wants to play the patient role (option C). **(pp. 264–266, 271)**

10.8   What is the recommended treatment for somatic symptom disorder?

A. Selective serotonin reuptake inhibitors (SSRIs).
B. Benzodiazepine tranquilizers.
C. Regularly scheduled visits with the same physician.
D. Referral to specialists in order to provide higher levels of care.
E. Aggressive workups to offer greater reassurance to patients.

The correct response is option C: Regularly scheduled visits with the same physician.

The recommendation is that patients with somatic symptom disorder have regularly scheduled visits with the same physician to provide reassurance and continuity of care (option C). This will reduce the likelihood that the patient will undergo unnecessary diagnostic studies and procedures (options D, E). Antidepressants (option A) have no established role in the treatment of somatic symptom disorders, with the possible exception of illness anxiety disorder. Long-term use of benzodiazepines (option B) is not recommended because of habituation and their abuse potential. **(pp. 273–275)**

10.9   A psychiatrist is asked to see a 25-year-old man with chronic renal failure admitted to a general medical floor for complications resulting from poor compliance with recommended dialysis. He shows a fair understanding of his medical condition but reports that he just feels like taking a day off from dialysis every now and again. Further interview doesn't reveal clear evidence of depression, anxiety, cognitive impairment, psychosis, or personality disorder. What is the most likely diagnosis?

A. Psychological factors affecting another medical condition.
B. Factitious disorder.
C. Malingering.
D. Unspecified depressive disorder.
E. Somatic symptom disorder.

The correct response is option A: Psychological factors affecting another medical condition.

The diagnosis in option A is used for patients without significant mental illness who otherwise have difficulty adhering to recommended medical treatments. Unlike a somatic symptom disorder (option E), these patients must have a clear medical diagnosis. Underlying psychological or behavioral factors include psychological distress, patterns of interpersonal interaction, coping styles, and maladaptive behaviors such as denial of symptoms or poor adherence to medical recommendations. Common examples are the person with anxiety exacerbating his or her asthma, denial of the need for treatment of acute chest pain, or manipulation of insulin by a person with diabetes wishing to lose weight. In this vignette, there is no evidence of motivation to play the patient role or for personal gain, making factitious disorder and malingering (options B, C) less likely. Option D is inappropriate because it is a diagnosis of exclusion. **(pp. 275–277)**

10.10 A psychiatrist is called to see a 25-year-old man with chronic renal failure admitted to a general medical floor for complications resulting from poor compliance with recommended dialysis. He has demanded to leave against medical advice. He has been threatening and verbally abusing staff members. He has fair understanding of his medical condition and is not delirious or confused. Review of his background shows a long history of legal and disciplinary problems dating to childhood. What is the best diagnosis?

A. Psychological factors affecting another medical condition.
B. Antisocial personality disorder.
C. Malingering.
D. Unspecified depressive disorder.
E. Somatic symptom disorder.

The correct response is option B: Antisocial personality disorder.

This patient's behavior should be diagnosed as a primary personality disorder (option B) rather than psychological factors affecting another medical condition (option A), which requires that the patient's behavior *not* be better explained by another mental disorder. There is no evidence of motivation to play the patient role or preoccupation with his somatic symptoms, ruling out malingering and somatic symptom disorder (options C, E). Option D is inappropriate because it is a diagnosis of exclusion. **(pp. 275–277)**

10.11   A 10-year-old boy receives a couple of new video games for his birthday. The following day he tells his mother that he does not feel up to going to school because of stomach upset, although he appears well. His mother gives him a thermometer to check his temperature and leaves the room. When she comes back, the thermometer shows a temperature of 112 degrees. What is the most likely diagnosis?

A. Factitious disorder.
B. Malingering.
C. Somatic symptom disorder.
D. Separation anxiety disorder.
E. Psychological factors affecting another medical condition.

The correct response is option B: Malingering.

The boy in this example is most likely feigning illness to stay home from school to play video games. Rubbing a thermometer (usually against a blanket or similar object) is one method used to fake a fever, although in this case the boy does not realize that 112 degrees is a preposterous temperature elevation! Feigning illness for personal gain constitutes malingering (option B). Feigning illness to occupy the sick role is consistent with factitious disorder (option A). There is no evidence to suggest the boy is avoiding school because of fear of parental separation, which would suggest a separation anxiety disorder (option D). Patients with somatic symptom disorder (option C) are preoccupied with one or more somatic symptoms present 6 or more months, symptoms that do not fit the vignette. The diagnosis of psychological factors affecting another medical condition (option E) requires the presence of a specific medical condition. **(pp. 264, 275, 277, 280)**

10.12 Which personality disorder is frequently comorbid with dissociative identity disorder?

    A. Schizotypal personality disorder.
    B. Schizoid personality disorder.
    C. Dependent personality disorder.
    D. Borderline personality disorder.
    E. Narcissistic personality disorder.

The correct response is option D: Borderline personality disorder.

Patients with dissociative identity disorder often meet criteria for other mental disorders. Borderline personality disorder, found in up to 70% of patients with dissociative identity disorder, is diagnosed on the basis of mood instability, identity disturbance, deliberate self-harm, and other symptoms characteristic of the disorder. **(p. 284)**

10.13 What is the standard treatment for depersonalization/derealization disorder?

    A. Benzodiazepine tranquilizers.
    B. Fluoxetine.
    C. Second-generation antipsychotic.
    D. Psychotherapy.
    E. There is no standard treatment for depersonalization/derealization disorder.

The correct response is option E: There is no standard treatment for depersonalization/derealization disorder.

There is no standard treatment for depersonalization/derealization disorder (option E). A controlled trial showed that fluoxetine (option B) was ineffective. Diazepam (option A) may lessen the anxiety that accompanies the disorder, but it is not a treatment for the disorder itself. While patients have been reported to benefit from cognitive-behavioral psychotherapy (option D) and hypnosis, these options are not considered standard treatments. There is no established role for antipsychotics in this condition (option C). **(pp. 289–290)**

10.14 A 19-year-old college student reports that for the past 2 weeks, since smoking cannabis for the first time, she has felt cut off from herself. She says that she feels she is watching herself go through the motions, and feels unable to connect with her experiences. She did not feel this way prior to smoking cannabis. What is the best diagnosis?

A. Dissociative identity disorder.
B. Depersonalization/derealization disorder.
C. Dissociative amnesia.
D. Substance-induced mood disorder.
E. Schizophrenia.

The correct response is option B: Depersonalization/derealization disorder.

Patients with depersonalization/derealization disorder feel disconnected from their experiences and/or surroundings (option B). This experience can occur in the course of another mental disorder, but the information provided in this vignette does not suggest one. Depersonalization/derealization disorder is sometimes preceded by the use of a substance such as marijuana, but substance-induced mood disorder (option D) is not an appropriate diagnosis because the complaints are of dissociation and not mood symptoms. Patients with dissociative identity disorder (option A) report feeling disconnected from reality, but this is due to their perception of having many personality states. Dissociative amnesia (option C) refers to the inability to recall important autobiographical information that is not attributable to ordinary forgetfulness. The patient is not reporting hallucinations or delusions, so schizophrenia is not a reasonable option (option E). **(pp. 281–282, 285, 288–289)**

10.15 A 35-year-old man presents to the emergency room. He shows the staff his driver's license and requests help because he has forgotten who he is and where he lives. His driver's license shows that he lives in a town over 100 miles away. A medical workup including brain imaging is unremarkable. Neuropsychological assessment shows gaps in his ability to recall autobiographical information, but formal testing of memory is normal. What is the most likely diagnosis?

A. Dissociative identity disorder.
B. Depersonalization/derealization disorder.
C. Dissociative amnesia.
D. Posttraumatic stress disorder.
E. Factitious disorder.

The correct response is option C: Dissociative amnesia.

The man is exhibiting a classic dissociative fugue, a diagnosis that is now classified in DSM-5 as a subtype ("with dissociative fugue") of dissociative amnesia (option C). The critical feature is that the person is unable to recall his past and assumes a new identity, which may be partial or complete. Fugues usually involve sudden, unexpected travel away from home or one's workplace, are not due to a dissociative identity disorder (option A), and are not induced by a substance or a general medical condition such as temporal lobe epilepsy. Fugue states are reported to occur in psychologically stressful situations, such as natural disasters, war, or personal rejections. Dissociative symptoms can occur in posttraumatic stress disorder but not in fugue states; furthermore, in posttraumatic stress disorder, the stressful event involves exposure to actual or threatened death (option D). The patient in this vignette is not feigning illness in order to play the patient role (option E), nor does he appear disconnected from his current experiences and/or surroundings (option B). **(pp. 285–288)**

—CHAPTER 11—

Feeding and Eating Disorders

11.1 A mother reports to a pediatrician that her 4-year-old son has been eating small quantities of dirt and pebbles from the garden at home. What is the most likely diagnosis?

A. Pica.
B. Rumination disorder.
C. Avoidant/restrictive food intake disorder.
D. Other specified feeding disorder.
E. None of the above.

The correct response is option A: Pica.

Pica is a pattern of eating nonnutritive substances on a persistent basis for at least 1 month (option A). Rumination disorder (option B) involves regurgitating swallowed food in the absence of a gastrointestinal disorder that would cause the disturbance. Patients with avoidant/restrictive food intake disorder (option C) have limited food intake rather than a propensity to eat nonnutritive substances. Option D is inappropriate because it is a diagnosis of exclusion. **(pp. 294–296)**

11.2 A mother reports to a pediatrician that her 15-month-old daughter mouths on a variety of inanimate objects in the home. What is the most likely diagnosis?

A. Pica.
B. Rumination disorder.

C. Avoidant/restrictive food intake disorder.
D. Other specified feeding disorder.
E. None of the above.

The correct response is option E: None of the above.

The daughter appears to be exhibiting normal developmental behavior in that she is mouthing objects and is under 2 years of age (option E). She does not fit the criteria for a more specific disorder or other specified feeding eating disorder (option D), nor is she swallowing regurgitated food (option B). Pica (option A) should not be diagnosed unless a child is over 2 years old. Patients with avoidant/restrictive food intake disorder (option C) have limited food intake rather than a propensity to eat nonnutritive substances. **(pp. 293–296)**

11.3. A 7-year-old child is brought to a pediatric gastroenterologist by her parents. They are concerned because they have noticed that the child has been regurgitating swallowed food, and then swallowing it again or sometimes expelling it. The child does not report symptoms such as heartburn or stomach pain. Her food intake is appropriate for her age, and she does not appear preoccupied with her body shape or size. A medical workup is unremarkable. What is the most likely diagnosis?

A. Pica.
B. Rumination disorder.
C. Avoidant/restrictive food intake disorder.
D. Bulimia nervosa.
E. Anorexia nervosa.

The correct response is option B: Rumination disorder.

The child has rumination disorder, which is characterized by the repeated regurgitation of food (option B). The disorder occurs across age ranges and in both genders. Individuals with this disorder repeatedly regurgitate swallowed or partially digested food, which may then be re-chewed and either reswallowed or expelled. Adolescents and adults are less likely to re-chew regurgitated material than younger children. This child does not have body image concerns that would characterize an eating disorder such as bulimia nervosa (option D) and anorexia nervosa (option E), or a pattern of restrictive or avoidance eating behavior (option C), and she is not ingesting nonnutritive substances (option A). **(pp. 294–301)**

11.4   An 11-year-old boy with autism spectrum disorder is brought to a pediatrician because his mother is concerned about his poor appetite. He has always been a picky eater, but his mother is especially concerned because it's about time for his "growth spurt." The boy is thin but not emaciated and is of normal height. He tells his doctor that he's not very interested in food and that he finds the textures of most foods unappetizing. He denies preoccupation with being thin, and there is no evidence of depression. What is the most likely diagnosis?

A. Pica.
B. Rumination disorder.
C. Avoidant/restrictive food intake disorder.
D. Bulimia nervosa.
E. Anorexia nervosa.

The correct response is option C: Avoidant/restrictive food intake disorder.

The boy in this case has an autism spectrum disorder and perhaps has unusual eating habits consistent with the restricted range of interests seen in such patients. That said, the key difference between avoidant/restrictive food intake disorder (option C) and an eating disorder such as anorexia nervosa or bulimia nervosa (options D, E) is that patients with avoidant/restrictive food intake disorder do not have preoccupation with their body image. Pica (option A) is a pattern of eating nonnutritive objects as food. Rumination disorder (option B) involves regurgitating swallowed food in the absence of a gastrointestinal disorder that would cause the disturbance. **(pp. 296–298)**

11.5   A 50-year-old man is brought to his family physician at his wife's insistence. She is concerned because he has lost 15 lbs. in the past month. He "barely eats a thing," she says. The man reports he no longer has any interest in anything. He spends most of the day watching TV but doesn't pay much attention to the programs. He complains of poor sleep, waking up at about 3 A.M. every morning and not being able to go back to sleep. He displays a restricted affect. What is the most likely diagnosis?

A. Pica.

B. Rumination disorder.

C. Avoidant/restrictive food intake disorder.

D. Major depressive disorder.

E. Anorexia nervosa.

The correct response is option D: Major depressive disorder.

The importance of this vignette is to highlight the fact that eating disturbances are common throughout psychiatry, and major depression is one of the main causes of poor appetite and weight loss. Thus, the patient's symptoms are consistent with a classic major depressive episode (option D) rather than a primary disorder of feeding or eating. This patient is not ingesting nonnutritive substances (option A), regurgitating swallowed food in the absence of a disorder that would cause the disturbance (option B), or engaging in disturbed eating patterns because of a preoccupation with his body weight and shape (option E). Avoidant/restrictive food intake disorder (option C) is not appropriate because the symptoms are better explained by major depressive disorder. **(pp. 167 [Chapter 6], 294–300)**

11.6   What is the key difference between anorexia nervosa and bulimia nervosa?

A. Presence of binging behavior.

B. Presence of purging behavior.

C. Preoccupation with one's body weight.

D. Current body weight.

E. Personality of the patient.

The correct response is option D: Current body weight.

Both disorders overlap and intertwine, but the fundamental difference is that patients with anorexia nervosa mainly restrict their food intake, whereas bulimic patients have episodes of binging eating and purging. Although patients with anorexia are significantly underweight, patients with bulimia tend to be of near-normal weight (option D), even when their illness is active. Both patients have an intense preoccupation with their body weight and shape (option C). Nonetheless, many anorexia patients have the binge-purge subtype (options A, B) and engage in significant binge eating followed by compensatory behaviors. Importantly, patients with anorexia and bulimia tend to have different personality characteristic personalities (option E), but this is not part of the DSM-5 diagnostic criteria. Bulimic patients more commonly have "acting out" personality disorders, such as borderline personality disorder, than do anorexia patients. **(pp. 298–308)**

11.7   Which of the following physical examination findings is *not* typical of anorexia nervosa?

A. Tachycardia.
B. Hypokalemia.
C. Amenorrhea.
D. Hair loss.
E. Constipation.

The correct response is option A: Tachycardia.

Patients with poorly controlled anorexia nervosa develop bradycardia rather than tachycardia (option A). Options B–E are common abnormalities. **(Table 11–2 [Medical complications of the eating disorders], p. 305)**

11.8   Which brain region plays an important role in regulating feeding behavior?

A. Thalamus.
B. Hypothalamus.
C. Pineal gland.
D. Amygdala.
E. Entorhinal cortex.

The correct response is option B: Hypothalamus.

The hypothalamus has a central role in regulating feeding behavior (option B). With the neurotransmitter serotonin, the hypothalamus helps modulate feeding behavior by producing feelings of fullness and satiety. It is unclear if the other regions listed in options A, C, D, and E play a role in eating disorders. **(p. 306)**

11.9   Which of the following physical examination findings would suggest a diagnosis of bulimia nervosa or the binge-purge subtype of anorexia nervosa rather than another eating disorder?

A. Constipation.

B. Decreased thyroid-stimulating hormone.

C. Calluses on the dorsal surface of the hands.

D. Amenorrhea.

E. Hair loss.

The correct response is option C: Calluses on the dorsal surface of the hands.

Patients who induce vomiting by inserting their fingers in their throat may develop calluses on the dorsal surfaces of their hands where the skin of their hands has contact with their teeth (option C). Options A, B, D, and E are not specific for purging behavior. **(p. 304)**

11.10 During a routine health maintenance exam, a 30-year-old man tells his family physician that he has been having trouble losing weight. He reports that 3–4 times each week, he loses control of his eating and consumes a very large quantity of food such that he feels physically uncomfortable afterward. He feels embarrassed, and because of this tendency he makes up excuses to reject dinner invitations. He is overweight and has some concern about his body image, but he denies being obsessed with being thin. He denies excessive exercise or other compensatory behaviors. What is the most likely diagnosis?

A. Binge-eating disorder.

B. Rumination disorder.

C. Avoidant/restrictive food intake disorder.

D. Bulimia nervosa.

E. Anorexia nervosa.

The correct response is option A: Binge-eating disorder.

The patient has a classic binge-eating disorder that is new to DSM-5 (option A). It is a diagnosis used for patients with recurrent spells of binge eating who do not have the compensatory behavior that is present in bulimia nervosa, such as purging (option D). Patients with avoidant/restrictive food intake disorder (option C) avoid eating and do not have binges. Patients with rumination disorder (option B) regurgitate swallowed food, but this is not a compensatory mechanism because these patients may re-swallow the regurgitated food and they do not have episodic binging be-havior. Many patients with binge-eating disorder are men, and most have a history of compensatory behaviors. Anorexia nervosa (option E) is not appropriate because there is no significant weight loss. **(pp. 301–302)**

11.11 Which antidepressant is contraindicated in patients with eating disorders?

A. Fluoxetine.
B. Sertraline.
C. Bupropion.
D. Venlafaxine.
E. Mirtazapine.

The correct response is option C: Bupropion.

Bupropion is contraindicated in patients with eating disorders because it can lower the seizure threshold in patients with electro-lyte disturbances. The other medications listed (options A, B, D, E) can be safely used in these patients. **(p. 309)**

11.12 Which medication is U.S. Food and Drug Administration (FDA) approved for the treatment of bulimia nervosa?

A. Sertraline.
B. Fluoxetine.
C. Lithium.
D. Venlafaxine.
E. Olanzapine.

The correct response is option B: Fluoxetine.

Fluoxetine is FDA approved for treatment of bulimia (option B). Other selective serotonin reuptake inhibitors (SSRIs), such as ser-traline (option A), and serotonin-norepinephrine reuptake inhib-itors, such as venlafaxine (option D), may be beneficial as well, but they have not been FDA approved for its treatment. Bupro-pion (option C) is contraindicated because it can lower the seizure threshold. Lithium (option C) and olanzapine (option E), a sec-ond-generation antipsychotic, have no role in the treatment of bulimia. **(pp. 309–310)**

11.13 What is the first objective in treating a patient with an eating disorder?

A. Correct faulty cognitions about body image.
B. Modify distorted eating behaviors.
C. Restore nutritional status.
D. Correct unhealthy home environment that gives rise to the disorder.
E. Initiate SSRI to address disrupted serotonergic neurotransmission.

The correct response is option C: Restore nutritional status.

In treating any patient with an eating disorder, the first order of business is to restore proper nutritional status (option C). This will help to correct electrolyte imbalances and restore a healthy body weight. The next objective is to modify disturbed eating behaviors (option B). The third objective is to correct cognitive distortions about body image (option A). SSRIs may help with bulimia nervosa, but they have no clear role in the treatment of anorexia (option E). Family and interpersonal therapy may be a helpful part of treatment, but these would fall under the second and third objectives (option D). **(pp. 308–310)**

CHAPTER 12

Sleep-Wake Disorders

12.1 Which sleep stage is characterized by rapid conjugate eye movements, penile/clitoral engorgement, and reduced muscle tone?

A. Stage 0.
B. Stage 1.
C. Stage 2.
D. Stage 3.
E. Rapid eye movement (REM) sleep.

The correct response is option E: Rapid eye movement (REM) sleep.

REM sleep is characterized by rapid conjugate eye movements, penile and clitoral engorgement, and reduced muscle tone (option E). Stage 0 sleep (option A) is wakefulness with eyes closed, characterized by alpha waves. Stage 1 sleep (option B) marks the transition from wakefulness to sleep, and it is characterized by beta and slow theta waves. Stage 2 sleep (option C) is characterized by the appearance of sleep spindles and K complexes. Stage 3 sleep (or deep sleep) (option D) is characterized by delta waves. **(p. 315)**

12.2 Which procedure can be used to measure excessive sleepiness?

A. Polysomnography.
B. Multiple Sleep Latency Test.
C. Electroencephalogram (EEG).
D. Clinical sleep hygiene assessment.
E. Neuropsychological evaluation.

The correct response is option B: Multiple Sleep Latency Test.

The Multiple Sleep Latency Test is used to measure excessive daytime sleepiness (option B). A patient is allowed an opportunity to fall asleep in a dark room for five 20-minute periods in 2-hour intervals. Polysomnography (option A) is the principal tool used to diagnose sleep disorders, including narcolepsy, parasomnias, and obstructive sleep apnea/hypopnea. EEG (option C) is a part of polysomnography. A clinical sleep hygiene assessment (option D) is an important part of evaluating sleep complaints but does not measure excessive sleepiness. A neuropsychological evaluation (option E) does not have a clearly defined role in the routine assessment of sleep disorders. **(p. 316)**

12.3 Which of the following is *not* a routine sleep hygiene recommendation?

A. Discontinuing the intake of alcohol, caffeine, and sedative-hypnotics.
B. Avoiding reading, working, or watching TV in bed.
C. Staying awake in bed for long periods of time until sleep onset occurs.
D. Going to bed and waking up at the same time every day, even on weekends.
E. Avoiding napping.

The correct response is option C: Staying awake in bed for long periods of time until sleep onset occurs.

Standard sleep hygiene recommends avoiding staying in bed awake for long periods of time (option C). Options A, B, D, and E are standard sleep hygiene recommendations. **(p. 319)**

12.4 Which of the following can be used to treat insomnia disorder?

A. Temazepam.
B. Trazodone.
C. Diphenhydramine.
D. Zolpidem.
E. All of the above.

The correct response is option E: All of the above.

Although improved sleep hygiene should be the starting point for the treatment of insomnia disorder, any of options A–D can be used. Hypnotics should be used to treat transient and short-term insomnia, in combination with appropriate sleep hygiene. **(pp. 319–320)**

12.5   A 35-year-old man complains to his family physician of difficulty falling asleep for the past 8 months. It takes him up to an hour to fall asleep, and he reports feeling fatigued throughout the day. He sometimes feels irritable but denies significant depression. He does not snore, nor does he feel sleepy during the day. He stopped his caffeine intake a couple of months ago after reading about sleep hygiene on the Internet. What is the most likely diagnosis?

A. Hypersomnolence disorder.
B. Narcolepsy.
C. Insomnia disorder.
D. Obstructive sleep apnea.
E. Other specified insomnia disorder.

The correct response is option C: Insomnia disorder.

The man in this vignette has an insomnia disorder, defined as trouble initiating or maintaining sleep on a regular basis for at least 3 months (option C). Comorbid psychiatric or medical problems do not preclude this diagnosis. Patients with hypersomnolence disorder (option A) do not feel rested in spite of excessive sleep. Patients with obstructive sleep apnea (option D) have frequent arousals secondary to hypoventilation, resulting in daytime sleepiness. Patients with narcolepsy (option B) have the recurrent irrepressible need to nap, decreased REM latency, hypocretin deficiency, and episodes of cataplexy. Other specified insomnia disorder (option E) is not appropriate because it is a diagnosis of exclusion. **(pp. 317–318, 320, 323, 326)**

12.6   Which of the following suggests hypersomnolence disorder rather than narcolepsy?

A. Daytime napping.
B. Decreased REM sleep latency.
C. Spells of brief loss of muscle tone (hypotonia).
D. Hypocretin deficiency.
E. Sleep inertia.

The correct response is option E: Sleep inertia.

Sleep inertia, or prolonged grogginess after waking, is more characteristic of hypersomnolence disorder than narcolepsy (option E). Daytime napping (option A) occurs in both disorders. Hypocretin deficiency (option D), decreased REM sleep latency (option B), and spells of hypotonia (option C) are characteristic of narcolepsy rather than hypersomnolence disorder. **(pp. 321–323)**

12.7   A 22-year-old woman presents to a sleep disorders clinic. She reports that she is groggy most every morning and it takes her over an hour to become alert. She sleeps 9–10 hours at night. She feels sleepy during the day and will sometimes take a 1- to 2-hour nap. She denies episodes of cataplexy or excessive caffeine use. Which treatment may be effective for this patient?

A. Selective serotonin reuptake inhibitor.
B. Benzodiazepine.
C. Stimulant.
D. Nonbenzodiazepine hypnotic.
E. Antihistamine.

The correct response is option C: Stimulant.

The woman in this vignette appears to have a hypersomnolence disorder, and stimulants such as methylphenidate are probably the most effective treatment (option C). They have the potential for abuse; therefore, their use needs careful monitoring. Improved sleep hygiene is also important. Scheduled napping may help as well. Antidepressants (option A) are not appropriate because there is no information to suggest that the patient is depressed. A benzodiazepine, a nonbenzodiazepine hypnotic, or an antihistamine (options B, D, E) would only cause greater sedation and are therefore inappropriate. **(p. 322)**

12.8   What causes narcolepsy?

A. Loss of cholinergic cells in the nucleus basalis.
B. Loss of hypocretin-secreting cells in the hypothalamus.
C. Decrease in REM latency.
D. Poor sleep hygiene.
E. The cause is unknown.

The correct response is option B: Loss of hypocretin-secreting cells in the hypothalamus.

Narcolepsy is one of the few DSM-5 disorders in which a biological mechanism has been identified (option E) and has been included in the criteria set. Narcolepsy nearly always results from the loss of hypothalamic hypocretin-producing cells (option B), causing cerebrospinal fluid hypocretin-1 deficiency (less than or equal to one-third of control values, or 110 pg/mL in most laboratories). (Hypocretin is a neurotransmitter that regulates arousal, wakefulness, and appetite.) As for the other response options, a decrease in REM latency (option C) is a symptom of narcolepsy rather than its cause. Poor sleep hygiene (option D) does not lead to narcolepsy. Loss of cholinergic cells in the nucleus basalis (option A) is a finding associated with Alzheimer's disease. **(pp. 323–325)**

12.9   Which of the following is an effective treatment for sleep attacks associated with narcolepsy?

A. Tricyclic antidepressant.
B. Sodium oxybate.
C. Methylphenidate.
D. Zolpidem.
E. Improved sleep hygiene.

The correct response is option C: Methylphenidate.

The clinical management of narcolepsy involves different treatments for the sleep attacks and the auxiliary symptoms. Stimulants such as methylphenidate (option C) or dextroamphetamine are the preferred drugs for treating sleep attacks because of their rapid onset and relative lack of side effects. Modafinil is an effective alternative to the stimulants. Sodium oxybate (option B) is U.S. Food and Drug Administration (FDA) approved for the treatment of cataplexy associated with narcolepsy and has been shown to reduce the frequency of cataplexy episodes. Tricyclic antidepressants (option A) are sometimes used to treat cataplexy or sleep paralysis but have little effect on sleep attacks. Zolpidem (option D) is an effective hypnotic but has no role in treating sleep attacks. Sleep hygiene (option C) should always be recommended to patients but will not treat sleep attacks. **(p. 325)**

12.10 What is the technical term used for a decrease in airflow during sleeping?

A. Apnea.
B. Hypopnea.
C. Hyperpnea.
D. Tachypnea.
E. Hyperpnoea.

The correct response is option B: Hypopnea.

Hypopnea (option B) is a decrease in airflow. Apnea (option A) is a pause in breathing. Tachypnea (option D) is an increase in the rate of breathing. Hyperpnea and hyperpnoea (options C, D) both refer to an increase in the depth of breathing. **(p. 326)**

12.11 A 45-year-old obese man complains to his family physician of chronic trouble with sleep maintenance. He falls asleep easily at night, but awakens 10–20 times throughout the night. He feels fatigued during the day and occasionally takes short naps. He says his wife tells him that he snores loudly at times but not on most nights. He sleeps in a quiet dark room and goes to bed at about the same time on most nights, but on the weekend he might stay up 30–45 minutes later than usual. His blood pressure is normal. He drinks 2–3 cups of coffee in the morning and may have a 12 oz. can of soda in the late afternoon. What is the best next step in management of this patient?

A. Prescribe a benzodiazepine.
B. Have the patient eliminate caffeine intake.
C. Administer Multiple Sleep Latency Test.
D. Administer polysomnogram.
E. Counsel the patient on sleep hygiene and follow-up in 3 months.

The correct response is option D: Administer polysomnogram.

The root cause of this patient's sleeping problems is not entirely clear, but obstructive sleep apnea needs to be ruled out with polysomnography (option D). Counseling the patient on sleep hygiene (option E) should also be done, but it is best to proceed with the polysomnography. Lifestyle changes alone are unlikely to have much of an impact, including eliminating caffeine intake (option B). If the patient has obstructive sleep apnea, a continuous positive airway pressure (CPAP) machine would be the method of choice to help him with sleep rather than a benzodiazepine (option A) or a hypnotic. The Multiple Sleep Latency Test (option C) measures daytime fatigue, but in this case polysomnography would provide more useful diagnostic information. **(pp. 316, 326–328)**

12.12 Which of the following is *not* suggestive of obstructive sleep apnea?

A. Snoring.
B. Daytime fatigue.
C. Apneic episodes.
D. Crescendo-decrescendo variation in tidal volume.
E. Difficulty to controlling hypertension.

The correct response is option D: Crescendo-decrescendo variation in tidal volume.

Crescendo-decrescendo variation in tidal volume is called *Cheyne-Stokes breathing*. This sort of breathing is characteristic of individuals who have central sleep apnea comorbid with heart failure, renal failure, or history of stroke. Options A–C and E are characteristics associated with obstructive sleep apnea. **(pp. 326–328)**

12.13 Which of the following treatment methods can be used for refractory cases of obstructive sleep apnea?

A. Weight-loss counseling.
B. Continuous positive airway pressure (CPAP).
C. Sedative-hypnotics.
D. Acetazolamide.
E. Uvulopalatopharyngoplasty.

The correct response is option E: Uvulopalatopharyngoplasty.

Uvulopalatopharyngoplasty is a surgical procedure used to correct refractory cases of obstructive sleep apnea (option E); patients who do not improve with this procedure may need a tracheostomy. Acetazolamide (option D) can be given to stimulate breathing in cases of central sleep apnea. Sedative-hypnotics (option C) should be avoided in obstructive sleep apnea. CPAP (option B) and weight-loss counseling (option A) are first-line treatments for obstructive sleep apnea. **(pp. 327–329)**

12.14 Which medication can be used to stimulate breathing in patients with central sleep apnea?

A. Sodium oxybate.
B. Chloral hydrate.
C. Acetazolamide.
D. Zolpidem.
E. Any benzodiazepine.

The correct response is option C: Acetazolamide.

Acetazolamide can be used to stimulate breathing in patients with central sleep apnea (option C). Theophylline can also be used. Sodium oxybate (option A) is used to treat cataplexy associated with narcolepsy. Chloral hydrate (option B), zolpidem (option D), and benzodiazepines (option E) can all depress respiration and have no role in the treatment of central sleep apnea. **(pp. 325, 329)**

12.15 A 50-year-old woman with chronic obstructive pulmonary disease reports to her family physician that she has morning headache and daytime fatigue. Routine laboratory studies are remarkable for elevated CO_2. Polysomnogram shows periods of decreased respiration. What is the most likely diagnosis?

A. Obstructive sleep apnea.
B. Central sleep apnea.
C. Sleep-related hypoventilation.
D. Hypersomnolence disorder.
E. Narcolepsy.

The correct response is option C: Sleep-related hypoventilation.

Sleep-related hypoventilation is the result of a decreased response to high carbon dioxide during sleep and is characterized by frequent episodes of shallow breathing lasting longer than 10 seconds during sleep (option C). Polysomnography shows episodes of decreased respiration associated with elevated CO_2 levels. It is usually associated with lung disease. Obstructive and central sleep apnea (options A, B) are characterized by episodes of apnea and hypopnea on a polysomnogram. Central sleep apnea is caused by variable respiratory effort and obstructive sleep apnea is caused by upper airway resistance. Patients with hypersomnolence disorder (option D) sleep excessively and still do not feel rested. Narcolepsy (option E) is characterized by sleep attacks and episodes of cataplexy. **(pp. 329–330)**

12.16 A 27-year-old man who works nights at a convenience store reports to his family physician that his energy is chronically low and he has little motivation. He can only sleep 4–6 hours during the day. He tries to maintain a diurnal schedule on his days off on the weekend but has trouble falling asleep at night. What is the most likely diagnosis?

A. Insomnia disorder.
B. Obstructive sleep apnea.
C. Hypersomnolence disorder.
D. Circadian rhythm sleep-wake disorder.
E. Narcolepsy.

The correct response is option D: Circadian rhythm sleep-wake disorder.

The man suffers from the shift work type of circadian rhythm sleep-wake disorder (option D). Shift workers tend to have high rates of on the job sleepiness, tend to make cognitive errors, and have high rates of drug use and divorce. They may never feel fully rested. When they want to sleep, they cannot, and when they are expected to be awake and alert, they are sleepy and drowsy. As for the other response options, insomnia disorder (option A) is trouble initiating or maintaining sleep on a regular basis for at least 3 months. Patients with hypersomnolence disorder (option C) do not feel rested in spite of excessive sleep. Patients with obstructive sleep apnea (option B) have frequent arousals secondary to hypoventilation, resulting in daytime sleepiness. Patients with narcolepsy (option E) have a recurrent, irrepressible need to nap, decreased REM latency, hypocretin deficiency, and episodes of cataplexy. **(pp. 331–333)**

12.17 What is the best treatment for circadian rhythm sleep-wake disorder, shift work type?

A. Improved sleep hygiene.
B. Methylphenidate to improve alertness.
C. Zolpidem to assist with daytime sleep.

D. Melatonin to regulate circadian rhythm.

E. Discontinue shift work.

The correct response is option E: Discontinue shift work.

Unfortunately, for the man in the vignette given above, the best option is to discontinue shift work (option E) and to resume a normal diurnal schedule. For most people, earning a paycheck often trumps such considerations. Although improved sleep hygiene could help, it cannot override the deleterious effect of shift change. Interestingly, the stimulant drug armodafinil has been FDA approved to treat shift work disorder. Options A–D will not help correct the man's sleep disorder. **(p. 333)**

12.18 What is the DSM-5 diagnosis used for both sleep walking and sleep terrors?

A. Non-REM (NREM) sleep arousal disorder.

B. REM sleep behavior disorder.

C. Parasomnia.

D. Circadian rhythm sleep-wake disorder.

E. None of the above.

The correct response is option A: NREM sleep arousal disorder.

Sleep walking and sleep terrors are both referred to as NREM sleep arousal disorders because they occur during stage 3 of sleep (option A). REM sleep behavior disorder (option B) occurs during REM sleep. Parasomnia (option C) is a general term used for abnormal behavior or experiences that occur during sleep or sleep-wake transitions. Circadian rhythm sleep-wake disorders (option D) are persistent or recurring patterns of sleep disruption that result from an altered sleep-wake schedule, or occur when the sleep-wake cycle is not correctly synchronized with a person's daily schedule. **(pp. 333–335)**

12.19 A 15-year-old boy has recurrent vivid dreams with frightening violent content. He wakes up in the morning with a racing heart and heavy breathing, but he does not scream or act out. What is the most likely diagnosis?

A. REM sleep behavior disorder.

B. NREM sleep arousal disorder, sleep terror type.

C. Nightmare disorder.
D. Parasomnia.
E. None of the above.

The correct response is option C: Nightmare disorder.

Nightmares are vivid, and patients may have some autonomic arousal upon awakening, but they do not scream upon awakening as do people with sleep terrors (option C). On a physiological level, nightmares occur during REM sleep (option B), whereas sleep terrors occur during NREM sleep. Parasomnia (option D) is a general term for abnormal experiences or behavior that occurs during sleep or sleep-wake transition. REM sleep behavior disorder (option A) is defined by the presence of arousal during REM sleep associated with vocalization and/or complex motor behaviors. **(pp. 336–337)**

12.20 Which sleep disorder is associated with Parkinson's disease, Lewy body dementia, and multiple systems atrophy?

A. REM sleep behavior disorder.
B. NREM sleep arousal disorder, sleep terror type.
C. Nightmare disorder.
D. Parasomnia.
E. Central sleep apnea.

The correct response is option A: REM sleep behavior disorder.

There is a relationship between REM sleep behavior disorder and neurodegenerative disorders (particularly Parkinson's disease, dementia with Lewy bodies, and multiple system atrophy). At least 50% of individuals with REM sleep behavior disorder presenting in sleep clinics will eventually develop one of these conditions. **(p. 338)**

12.21 A 31-year-old woman reports to her family physician that she has the uncomfortable sensation of having to move her legs at night when she is in bed. She says she does not sleep well because of this. She wonders if something can be given to treat her condition. Which of the following can be used to treat this condition?

A. Zolpidem.
B. Pramipexole.

C. L-Dopa.
D. Clonazepam.
E. Imipramine.

The correct response is option B: Pramipexole.

The woman has restless legs syndrome, which is now classified as a sleep-wake disorder in DSM-5 because it interferes with sleep and may be associated with periodic limb movements during sleep. The syndrome affects about 5% of the general population. Patients report that symptoms begin in the evening and are relieved by moving the legs or walking. The sensations can delay sleep or waken the person from sleep. Dopamine agonists such as pramipexole or ropinirole may be used to treat restless legs syndrome (option B). Curiously, these drugs have been alleged to induce compulsive behaviors such as gambling, shopping, and even sex. Physicians need to be alert to these possible complications and ask their patients about them. Options A, D, and E are not treatments for restless legs syndrome. L-Dopa (option C) can be used, but it is a second-line choice because of its many side effects. **(pp. 339–340)**

CHAPTER 13

Sexual Dysfunction, Gender Dysphoria, and Paraphilias

13.1   How long should a disorder of sexual function be present prior to diagnosis?

   A. At least 18 months.
   B. At least 4 months.
   C. At least 1 month.
   D. At least 6 months.
   E. At least 1 year.

The correct response is option D: At least 6 months.

DSM-5 requires that disorders of sexual function be present for a minimum duration of at least 6 months prior to diagnosis. **(p. 345)**

13.2   Which of the following would preclude a diagnosis of a sexual dysfunction?

   A. Severe relationship stress.
   B. A nonsexual mental disorder that would account for symptoms.
   C. Disturbance caused by substance use or medication.
   D. Disturbance caused by medical condition such as diabetes.
   E. Any of the above would preclude diagnosis.

The correct response is option E: Any of the above would preclude diagnosis.

Any of the items listed would preclude a diagnosis of a sexual dysfunction (option E). DSM-5 requires that in addition to having persisted 6 months or longer, the disorder causes clinically significant distress. DSM-5 requires further that the disorder is not due to severe relationship stress, another nonsexual mental disorder, or to the effects of a substance, medication, or medical condition (options A–D) (e.g., diabetes mellitus). **(p. 345)**

13.3   A 22-year-old man reports to his family physician that he has had persistent difficulty achieving orgasm during intercourse with his partner. He has no trouble attaining an erection. The problem has been ongoing since the relationship began about a year ago. He does not have any difficulty achieving orgasm during masturbation and reports that otherwise his relationship is going well. He does not take any medications. What is the most likely diagnosis?

A. No diagnosis.
B. Other specified sexual dysfunction.
C. Delayed ejaculation.
D. Male hypoactive sexual desire disorder.
E. Erectile disorder.

The correct response is option C: Delayed ejaculation.

The fact that the problem only occurs during intercourse with a partner does not preclude a diagnosis of delayed ejaculation (option C). The patient denies problems achieving an erection, ruling out erectile disorder (option E), and nothing in the vignette indicates a problem with sexual desire (option D). The patient's difficulty as described does meet criteria for a more specific sexual dysfunction (option B). **(pp. 343, 346–347)**

13.4   A 28-year-old man reports to his family physician that he has had persistent difficulty achieving orgasm both with his partner and while masturbating. He has no trouble attaining an erection. His problem has been ongoing since the relationship began about a year ago. He reports that otherwise his relationship is going well. He does not take any medications except for fluoxetine. What is the most likely diagnosis?

A. Medication-induced sexual dysfunction.
B. Other specified sexual dysfunction.

C. Delayed ejaculation.
D. Male hypoactive sexual desire disorder.
E. Erectile disorder.

The correct response is option A: Medication-induced sexual dysfunction.

Fluoxetine, along with the other selective serotonin reuptake inhibitors (SSRIs), can induce sexual dysfunction (option A). Typically, this consists of ejaculatory delay or failure in men. The vignette indicates no difficulty with ejaculation or desire or occurrence of erectile difficulty (options C–E). Other specified sexual disorder (option B) is inappropriate because it is a diagnosis of exclusion. **(pp. 355–357, 359)**

13.5   A 40-year-old man with type 2 diabetes mellitus reports to his family physician that he has progressive difficulty achieving an erection prior to intercourse with his wife. He continues to experience spontaneous erections at times when he is not planning to have intercourse. What is the most likely etiology of the patient's problem?

A. Secondary to type 2 diabetes mellitus.
B. Secondary to psychological factors.
C. Secondary to marital discord.
D. Secondary to a medical condition other than type 2 diabetes.
E. Unable to determine without more information.

The correct response is option B: Secondary to psychological factors.

The presence of spontaneous erections would suggest a psychological origin of erectile dysfunction despite the presence of type 2 diabetes mellitus. In determining the cause, it is important to determine whether spontaneous erections occur at times when the man does not plan to have intercourse (e.g., morning erections, erections with masturbation). If erections occur at these times, the disorder is more likely to have a psychological origin (option B). **(pp. 357–359)**

13.6   A 30-year-old woman reports to her family physician of ongoing sexual difficulties with her partner for the last several years. She experiences vaginal and pelvic pain during intercourse. She denies that there is difficulty achieving vaginal penetration, and she is not sure about tightening of her pelvic muscles during penetration. What is the most likely diagnosis?

A. Dyspareunia.
B. Vaginismus.
C. Genito-pelvic pain disorder.
D. Female sexual interest/arousal disorder.
E. None of the above.

The correct response is option C: Genito-pelvic pain disorder.

Genito-pelvic pain disorder is diagnosed when a person has pain or discomfort, muscular tightening, or fear about pain when having sexual intercourse (option C). This disorder reflects a change from DSM-IV, wherein two disorders—dyspareunia and vaginismus (options A, B)—were used to diagnose sexual pain disorders. They are now merged into a single category because clinicians had difficulty in distinguishing between the two, and their reliability was low. Female sexual interest/arousal disorder (option D) reflects a decreased interest in sexual activity rather than pain and difficulty with vaginal penetration. **(pp. 350–352)**

13.7 A 50-year-old man reports to his family physician that in the past few months he has had a new onset of premature ejaculation during intercourse. He is baffled about why it is happening at his age. He has been feeling more jittery than usual over the past few months, and he reports occasional palpitations and diaphoresis on review of systems. What is the next best step in management of this patient?

A. Refer to a psychiatrist.
B. Start a selective serotonin reuptake inhibitor (SSRI).
C. Refer to a psychotherapist.
D. Order thyroid-stimulating hormone.
E. None of the above.

The correct response is option D: Order thyroid-stimulating hormone.

Hyperthyroidism can cause late-onset premature ejaculation, and the patient's other symptoms suggest hyperthyroidism as well (option D). Options A–C would not be constructive in uncovering the underlying etiology for the patient's complaint. **(pp. 357–358)**

13.8   What medication can be used to treat premature ejaculation?

   A. Sildenafil.
   B. Alprostadil.
   C. Vardenafil.
   D. Paroxetine.
   E. Tadalafil.

The correct response is option D: Paroxetine.

Medication has assumed an increasing role in the treatment of the sexual dysfunctions. Paroxetine (option D) and other SSRIs can be used to treat premature (early) ejaculation because a common side effect is ejaculatory delay. Men can also benefit from 1% dibucaine (Nupercaine) ointment applied to the coronal ridge and frenulum of the penis to reduce stimulation. Options A–C and E are used to treat erectile disorder. **(p. 360)**

13.9   Which of the following medications is a standard treatment for erectile disorder?

   A. Vardenafil.
   B. Paroxetine.
   C. Dibucaine.
   D. Testosterone.
   E. Topical estrogen.

The correct response is option A: Vardenafil.

Vardenafil is one of the phosphoesterase-5 inhibitors, which are the first-line treatment for erectile disorder (option A). Paroxetine and dibucaine (options B, C) can be used to treat premature ejaculation. Testosterone (option D) is sometimes given for low sexual desire, but unless it is being used to treat hypogonadism, the results are mixed. Men should not be given topical estrogen (option E). **(p. 359)**

13.10 Which of the following is *not* typical of gender dysphoria?

A. Onset occurs in childhood.
B. The child prefers to play with children of the same gender.
C. The child expresses a strong desire to be rid of one's primary and secondary sexual characteristics because of incongruence between one's expressed and experienced gender.
D. The child expresses strong preference for cross-sex roles in make-believe play.
E. The child shows a strong preference for games, toys, and activities stereotypically associated with the opposite gender.

The correct response is option B: The child prefers to play with children of the same gender.

In childhood, patients with gender dysphoria generally prefer to play with children of the opposite gender (option B). Options A, C–E are typical of gender dysphoria. **(p. 362)**

13.11 A 40-year-old man reports to his psychiatrist that he enjoys dressing in women's clothing prior to intercourse, but this has caused conflict with his wife. He identifies himself as heterosexual, and he reports he is comfortable being male. What is the best diagnosis?

A. Gender dysphoria.
B. Transvestic disorder.
C. Voyeuristic disorder.
D. Exhibitionistic disorder.
E. Frotteuristic disorder.

The correct response is option B: Transvestic disorder.

Transvestic disorder is a paraphilia in which one becomes sexually aroused by dressing in the clothes of the opposite gender (option B). Patients with gender dysphoria (option A), in contrast, experience distress because of a perceived incongruence between their assigned and experienced genders. Patients with voyeuristic disorder (option C) become aroused by watching unsuspecting individuals when disrobing, naked, or engaged in sexual activity. Exhibitionistic disorder (option D) involves becoming aroused by exposing one's genitals to unsuspecting individuals, and frotteuristic disorder (option E) involves becoming sexually aroused from rubbing against a nonconsenting individual. **(pp. 368–370)**

13.12 What is the DSM-5 term for an anomalous sexual activity preference?

A. Paraphilic disorder.
B. Paraphilia.
C. Infantilism.
D. Infantilism disorder.
E. None of the above.

The correct response is option B: Paraphilia.

Paraphilia is the term used to describe anomalous sexual activity preference (option B). Paraphilic disorder (option A) refers to the distress experienced because of an anomalous sexual activity preference. Infantilism (option C) is a paraphilia in which the person obtains sexual arousal and gratification by behaving like an infant. Infantilism disorder (option D) is not a DSM-5 disorder. Infantilism should be coded as other specified paraphilic disorder. **(pp. 364–365)**

13.13 What is the standard treatment for paraphilic disorders?

A. SSRI.
B. Leuprolide.
C. Naltrexone.
D. Cognitive-behavioral therapy.
E. Medroxyprogesterone.

The correct response is option D: Cognitive-behavioral therapy.

Cognitive-behavioral therapy is the treatment mainstay for paraphilic disorders (option D). There are no medications U.S. Food and Drug Administration approved for paraphilic disorders (options A–C), but the medications listed have the goal of reducing paraphilic fantasies and behavior. The testosterone-lowering agents are generally reserved for patients with recurring legal problems that have resulted from a paraphilic disorder and may present a danger to the public. **(pp. 370–371)**

─ CHAPTER 14 ─

Disruptive, Impulse-Control, and Conduct Disorders

14.1 A 7-year-old girl is brought to a therapist by her mother. Her mother says that the girl is always touchy and irritable and gets very angry when she is told to do anything. The behavior has been present for over a year. When asked about her symptoms, the girl says that it's her mother's fault for always making her mad. She has not engaged in any stealing, fire setting, or runaway behavior. She gets along with her peers, and her grades in school are good. What is the most likely diagnosis?

A. Antisocial personality disorder.
B. Conduct disorder.
C. Attention deficit/hyperactivity disorder.
D. Oppositional defiant disorder.
E. Normal development.

The correct response is option D: Oppositional defiant disorder.

Oppositional defiant disorder is characterized by irritable, angry, and defiant behavior that does not involve frank antisocial behavior (option D). Antisocial personality disorder (option A) is a diagnosis reserved for adults; children with antisocial behavior receive a diagnosis of conduct disorder (option B). Nothing in the vignette suggests attention-deficit/hyperactivity disorder (option C). Whereas most children are occasionally naughty, children with oppositional defiant disorder are more frequently naughty, and more so than most children at the same mental age (option E). (pp. 376–378)

14.2   A 16-year-old boy with an autism spectrum disorder is brought to the emergency room by his family. His father reports that he broke two windows and smashed several plates in the kitchen after his father told him that he would not be able to use the computer for the next day because he had failed to clean up his room. The boy has had similar destructive outbursts when his computer privileges have been restricted in the past. Ordinarily, he is quiet, keeps to himself, and does not bother others. He does not have a history of truancy, fire setting, cruelty to animals, or fighting. What is the most likely diagnosis?

A. Oppositional defiant disorder.
B. Conduct disorder.
C. Antisocial personality disorder.
D. Intermittent explosive disorder.
E. No additional diagnosis apart from autism spectrum disorder.

The correct response is option D: Intermittent explosive disorder.

Intermittent explosive disorder can be diagnosed in addition to an autism spectrum disorder if the outbursts are significant enough to merit clinical attention (option D). It appears that the outburst is not typical behavior for this child and only occurs in a circumscribed context, making oppositional defiant disorder and conduct disorder (options A, B) less credible diagnostic options. Antisocial personality disorder (option C) is a diagnosis reserved for adults. (pp. 379–381)

14.3   A 16-year-old boy is brought to a psychiatrist at his parents' insistence for problem behavior ongoing for 3 years. He has had repeated legal trouble for acts of vandalism, and he has been expelled from school several times for fighting. He is failing all of his classes. He tells the psychiatrist that he doesn't care about his school work and has no remorse for his actions. What DSM-5 specifier is appropriate for this form of conduct disorder?

A. With limited prosocial emotions.
B. With antisocial personality features.
C. With psychopathic personality features.

D. Childhood-onset type.

E. DSM-5 does not have a descriptor for such cases.

The correct response is option A: With limited prosocial emotions.

"Limited prosocial emotions" is the DSM-5 specifier used for children with conduct disorder who show no remorse or interest in meeting societal expectations (option A). This is the childhood equivalent of psychopathy. He would qualify for the specifier adolescent onset type but not childhood-onset type (option D), which is for children whose conduct disorder has an onset prior to age 10 years. Options B and C are terms that are not used in DSM-5. **(pp. 381–383)**

14.4   A 35-year-old man is charged with arson after burning down a building he owned in order to collect insurance money. He has no previous criminal history, and his work history has been stable. He denies any previous episodes of fire setting. What is the most likely psychiatric diagnosis?

A. Antisocial personality disorder.

B. Adult antisocial behavior.

C. Pyromania.

D. Intermittent explosive disorder.

E. Conduct disorder.

The correct response is option B: Adult antisocial behavior.

The man's action appears to be criminal activity that has occurred in the absence of a specific mental disorder. Persons with antisocial personality disorder (option A) and conduct disorder (option E) have an enduring pattern of antisocial behavior, and a single action is inconsistent with these constructs. Patients with pyromania (option C) have a recurrent compulsion to set fires, and they are not typically motivated by material gain. In DSM-5, adult antisocial behavior is classified as a "V/Z code" diagnosis, that is, a condition that may be a focus of clinical attention but is not considered a mental disorder (option B). Intermittent explosive disorder (option D) is associated with recurrent behavioral outbursts, but that would not explain the man's behavior. **(pp. 280 [Chapter 10], 386)**

14.5   What is the treatment for pyromania?

A. Cognitive-behavioral therapy.
B. Selective serotonin reuptake inhibitor (SSRI).
C. Mood stabilizer such as carbamazepine.
D. Atypical antipsychotic such as risperidone.
E. There is no standard treatment for pyromania.

The correct response is option E: There is no standard treatment for pyromania.

There is no standard treatment for pyromania. Clinicians should begin by identifying other co-occurring mental disorders that can be a focus of treatment, such as major depression. Treatment of the co-occurring disorder may itself reduce fire-setting behavior. There is no clear role for medication in the treatment of pyromania. If the patient is a child or adolescent, the parents should be taught consistent but nonpunitive methods of discipline. Family therapy may help in dealing with the broader issue of family dysfunction often found in patients with pyromania. The patient needs to understand the dangerousness and significance of the fire setting. **(p. 387)**

14.6   A 24-year-old woman comes forward to establish care with a therapist. She reports a problem with compulsive stealing. She has taken small items of modest value from stores and from the homes of friends and family on many occasions since adolescence. She reports feeling tension before the theft and a sense of gratification afterward. She is motivated to change her behavior because she was recently given probation as a consequence of shoplifting. She denies any other criminal activity or interpersonal problems. What is the most likely diagnosis?

A. Conduct disorder.
B. Antisocial personality disorder.
C. Kleptomania.
D. Adult antisocial behavior.
E. Oppositional defiant disorder.

The correct response is option C: Kleptomania.

Kleptomania is compulsive stealing of objects of modest value (option C), and the stealing behavior does not occur in the context of a wider pattern of antisocial behavior as in conduct disorder (option A), a diagnosis applicable to children and adolescents, and antisocial personality disorder (option B). Adult antisocial behavior (option D) would be a reasonable option if the behavior were not accompanied by feelings of tension buildup before stealing followed by a sense of gratification. Oppositional defiant disorder (option E) is a diagnosis for children who are irritable, defiant, and quick to anger but who do not regularly engage in behavior that infringes upon the rights of others. **(pp. 387–388)**

14.7 All but which of the following may be beneficial for patients with intermittent explosive disorder?

A. Fluoxetine.
B. Oxcarbazepine.
C. Cognitive-behavior therapy.
D. Benzodiazepine tranquilizers.
E. Fluoxetine and oxcarbazepine.

The correct response is option D: Benzodiazepine tranquilizers.

Benzodiazepines should be avoided because of their tendency to cause behavioral disinhibition (option D). Both fluoxetine (option A) and the antiepileptic drug oxcarbazepine (option B), and their combination (option E), have been found superior to placebo in reducing impulsive aggression in people with intermittent explosive disorder. Other SSRIs, mood stabilizers, and β-blockers have been used to treat the condition, but their use is supported mainly by case studies or small case series. Second-generation antipsychotics have been used to dampen aggressive impulses in other clinical populations and may be helpful in treating intermittent explosive disorder, but they have not been specifically studied. Cognitive-behavioral therapy may be helpful (option C). **(p. 380)**

14.8 Naltrexone has shown to be more effective than placebo for treating which of the following?

A. Intermittent explosive disorder.
B. Conduct disorder.
C. Kleptomania.
D. Pyromania.
E. Oppositional defiant disorder.

The correct response is option C: Kleptomania.

There are no standard treatments for kleptomania, but medication may be helpful in some patients (option C). Naltrexone has specifically be found more effective than placebo in a randomized controlled trial, but it requires careful monitoring and can cause nausea and vomiting. SSRI antidepressants have also been used to treat the disorder. **(p. 388)**

—CHAPTER 15—

Substance-Related and Addictive Disorders

15.1   A 48-year-old woman reports to her family physician that she has been drinking a bottle of wine two to three times per week for the past 3 years. She has not been successful in her attempts to cut back her drinking, and her drinking has led to conflicts with her family. She has not had any problems at work as the result of her drinking, and she has never had symptoms of alcohol withdrawal. What is the best diagnosis?

A. Alcohol use disorder.
B. Alcohol dependence.
C. Alcohol abuse.
D. Alcoholism.
E. Alcohol abuse disorder.

The correct response is option A: Alcohol use disorder.

Alcohol use disorder is the new DSM-5 disorder that merges the DSM-IV-TR disorders of alcohol dependence and alcohol abuse (options B, C). Neither alcoholism nor alcohol abuse disorder (options D, E) is a DSM-IV-TR or DSM-5 diagnosis. Alcohol use disorder (option A) is further specified as mild, moderate, or severe, depending on the number of symptoms present. These diagnostic changes apply to all substance use disorders. **(pp. 392– 394)**

15.2 How long can cannabis be detected by urine drug screen after last use?

A. 24 hours.
B. 3 days.
C. 1 week.
D. 3 weeks.
E. 6 weeks.

The correct response is option D: 3 weeks.

Cannabis is fat soluble and can be detected on urine drug screen up to 3 weeks after last use. **(p. 395)**

15.3 Which neurotransmitter plays a key role in the development of all substance use disorders?

A. Serotonin.
B. Acetylcholine.
C. β-Endorphin.
D. Norepinephrine.
E. Dopamine.

The correct response is option E: Dopamine.

Research has begun to identify the neurobiologic substrates of addiction. Dopamine pathways that form part of the central nervous system "reward system" have been identified in the ventral tegmental region of the forebrain and in the nucleus accumbens. All drugs of abuse appear to target the brain's reward system by flooding the circuit with dopamine. **(p. 396)**

15.4 Which neurotransmitter plays a role specifically in the development of opioid use disorders?

A. Dopamine.
B. β-Endorphin.
C. Acetylcholine.
D. Serotonin.
E. Norepinephrine.

The correct response is option B: β-Endorphin.

Opioids activate μ receptors that release β-endorphins (option B), the chemical that is released when human beings engage in naturally rewarding activities (e.g., eating, sex). Dopamine (option A) modulates the reward system and is important in the development of all substance use disorders, but its importance is not specific to opioid use disorders. Acetylcholine (option C) has a major role in mediating memory. Serotonin (option D) has a role in modulating mood, anxiety, and aggression. Norepinephrine (option E) has a role in mediating the mood disorders. **(p. 396)**

15.5   A 17-year-old girl is referred for treatment of substance misuse. She smokes cannabis nearly every day and has started to use cocaine a few times a week in the past 2 months. Her father drinks excessively, and the family receives government assistance. One reason she gives for using illegal drugs is that her friends use these substances, and it is hard for her not to go along with them. Which of the following factors associated with this patient is *not* associated with risk of developing a substance use disorder?

A. Low socioeconomic status.
B. Susceptibility to peer influence.
C. Female sex.
D. Age.
E. Parental alcoholism.

The correct response is option C: Female sex.

The girl in the vignette unfortunately has many risk factors for substance misuse, which does not bode well for her future. That said, female sex is less likely to predispose to a substance use disorder than male sex (option C). Options A, B, D, and E are all factors are associated with risk of developing a substance use disorder. **(pp. 391–397)**

15.6   How many positive responses on a CAGE test are needed to indicate that a person may have an alcohol use disorder?

A. One.
B. Two.
C. Three.
D. Four.
E. The CAGE test is not a good screening test for alcohol use disorders.

The correct response is option A: One.

Even one positive response or overly defensive answer on the CAGE test, a simple screen that can be used to assess the presence of an alcohol use disorder, can indicate problematic use. A positive screen should be followed up with more detailed discussion. **(p. 399, Table 15–2 [CAGE: screening test for an alcohol use disorder], p. 400)**

15.7   Which of the following develops as a late-stage consequence of an alcohol use disorder?

A. Decreased work productivity.
B. Moodiness or irritability.
C. Palmar erythema.
D. Rosacea.
E. Jaundice.

The correct response is option E: Jaundice.

Jaundice develops in the later stages of alcohol use disorder and indicates advanced liver disease. The symptoms in options A–D develop earlier in the course. **(pp. 400–401)**

15.8   A 45-year-old man reports a 10-year history of heavy alcohol consumption to his family physician. He tells his physician that he is not as "sharp" as he used to be before he started drinking and that he has some mild difficulties with everyday memory tasks. He asks his doctor if these memory problems will be permanent. What is the best response?

A. "Even if you stop drinking, these memory problems are likely to be irreversible but not progressive."
B. "Even if you stop drinking, these memory problems are likely to be irreversible and progressive."
C. "If you stop drinking now, these memory problems may partially reverse."
D. "If you stop drinking now, your memory will likely fully completely."
E. None of the above.

The correct response is option C: "If you stop drinking now, these memory problems may partially reverse."

The physician can feel comfortable in sharing the good news: Neuropsychological testing of alcoholic persons generally reveals mild to moderate cognitive deficits that partially reverse with sobriety. Chronic alcohol misuse also has been associated with enlarged cerebral ventricles and widened cortical sulci—effects that also may be partially reversible if the individual stops drinking. **(p. 402)**

15.9   What percentage of motor vehicle deaths are related to alcohol?

A. 10%.
B. 20%.
C. 30%.
D. 40%.
E. >50%.

The correct response is option E: >50%.

More than 50% of motor vehicle deaths are related to alcohol. **(p. 403)**

15.10 Which of the following are the last symptoms to develop during the course of severe alcohol withdrawal?

A. Delirium, fever, autonomic hyperarousal.
B. Auditory, visual, tactile hallucinations in the presence of a clear sensorium.
C. Seizures.
D. Anxiety, tremor, nausea.
E. Increased heart rate and blood pressure.

The correct response is option A: Delirium, fever, autonomic hyperarousal.

Alcohol withdrawal delirium, which includes fever and autonomic hyperarousal, develops 2–3 days after cessation or major reduction in drinking behavior (option A). The first symptoms to develop are anxiety, tremor, nausea, and increased heart rate and blood pressure (options D, E). These symptoms develop 6–24 hours after cessation or reduction in drinking. Seizures (option C) occur from 7 hours up to 2 days after cessation or reduction in drinking. Hallucinations (option B) can occur within 48 hours and can last for up to a week. **(pp. 404–405)**

15.11 A psychiatrist is called to evaluate a 38-year-old man for admission to a psychiatric unit for alcohol detoxification and treatment of depression. He has been drinking large quantities of vodka daily for several months. He previously drank 3–4 beers nearly daily for almost 5 years. His last drink was 6 hours ago. He is currently pleasant and cooperative. His is fully oriented and in no distress. The psychiatrist asks the man if he has ever had the delirium tremens. He responds, "Oh yeah, I've got the shakes right now," and he holds out his hands to show the psychiatrist his mild tremor. How shall the psychiatrist proceed?

A. Recommend admission to intensive care because delirium tremens (DTs) can be fatal.
B. Admit the patient to psychiatry for alcohol rehabilitation.
C. Administer chlordiazepoxide now.
D. Collect additional information such as if the man has ever had confusion and fever during withdrawal or had become agitated.
E. None of the above.

The correct response is option D: Collect additional information such as if the man has ever had confusion and fever during withdrawal or had become agitated.

Many patients (and physicians) do not know what constitutes alcohol withdrawal delirium and will confuse tremors that develop during the earliest part of withdrawal with DTs. In these cases, the psychiatrist should collect additional information to determine if the patient has ever had an alcohol withdrawal delirium episode (option D). Patients at risk for severe withdrawal symptoms may require supportive care on a medical-surgical unit or intensive care unit (option A). Disposition is best decided after information gathering is complete. Administering chlordiazepoxide (option C) or another benzodiazepine should be started, but this response option does not address the issue of patient disposition. Alcohol rehabilitation (option B) will be important later, but the man first needs to be withdrawn from alcohol while being medically monitored. **(p. 405)**

15.12 Which medication used to treat alcohol dependence works by inhibiting alcohol dehydrogenase?

A. Naltrexone.
B. Disulfiram.

C. Acamprosate.

D. Chlordiazepoxide.

E. Lorazepam.

The correct response is option B: Disulfiram.

Disulfiram inhibits alcohol dehydrogenase, leading to the accumulation of acetaldehyde if the patient consumes alcohol, causing symptoms such as flushing, nausea, and vomiting to occur (option B). Naltrexone (option A) is a μ-opioid antagonist and reduces cravings. Acamprosate (option C) is a glutamate receptor modulator that reduces cravings. Chlordiazepoxide and lorazepam (options D, E) are benzodiazepines that can be used to treat acute alcohol withdrawal. **(pp. 406–409)**

15.13 A 20-year-old student sees his internist for anxiety symptoms. He reports that he has started worrying about everything since he started college about 2 years ago. He has trouble falling asleep and staying asleep nearly every night. His mood is mildly irritable, and he appears restless. He does not smoke, use alcohol, or use illicit drugs. He reports that he drinks eight or more cups of coffee daily to help him stay motivated when studying, with his last cup around 8–10 P.M. What is the most likely diagnosis?

A. Generalized anxiety disorder.

B. Bipolar I disorder.

C. Caffeine-induced anxiety disorder.

D. Panic disorder.

E. Insomnia disorder.

The correct response is option C: Caffeine-induced anxiety disorder.

Caffeine can cause or exacerbate anxiety disorders. Given this patient's excessive caffeine intake, caffeine-induced anxiety disorder is the best diagnosis (option C). Should he still complain of continued anxiety after significantly reducing his caffeine intake, generalized anxiety disorder (option A) would be a reasonable consideration. Irritability and insomnia in themselves are not sufficient to diagnose a manic episode associated with a bipolar disorder (option B). Panic attacks are acute spells of severe anxiety that last 15–20 minutes; therefore, panic disorder (option D) does not fit the pattern described in the vignette. Insomnia disorder (option E) would be a credible option if there was no history of excessive caffeine intake. **(pp. 410–411)**

15.14 Which of the following is *not* associated with cannabis use?

A. Increased risk of developing schizophrenia.
B. Increased risk of smoking cigarettes and abusing other drugs.
C. Tachycardia, dry mouth, and conjunctivitis during intoxication.
D. Flashbacks between periods of use.
E. Feeling that time has slowed and increased appetite during intoxication.

The correct response is option D: Flashbacks between periods of use.

Flashbacks between periods of use are associated with hallucinogens such as lysergic acid diethylamide (LSD) (option D). Options A–C and E are associated with cannabis use. **(pp. 411–412)**

15.15 A 19-year-old man presents to the emergency room complaining of acute-onset severe anxiety, confusion, time expansion, and vivid visual hallucinations. He took LSD for the first time 3 hours ago and is very uncomfortable, but he is cooperative in interview. His pupils are dilated, and he has mild tachycardia. Reassurance does not succeed in calming him down. What is the next best step in managing this case?

A. Give an antipsychotic.
B. Give a benzodiazepine.
C. Give clonidine.
D. Give naltrexone.
E. Refer the man to a substance use treatment program.

The correct response is option B: Give a benzodiazepine.

The man is experiencing a "bad trip" from LSD. Benzodiazepines can be used to calm patients who develop severe anxiety secondary to hallucinogen intoxication (option B). Clonidine (option C) can be used to help patients through opioid withdrawal. Naltrexone (option D) is one alternative to help patients with opioid use disorders maintain abstinence. An antipsychotic (option A) may be necessary to calm a patient who develops agitation secondary to phencyclidine or stimulant use. Although this patient would benefit from some form of substance use disorder treatment, such a referral would not address his immediate report of anxiety secondary to acute hallucinogen intoxication (option E). **(p. 414, 418–419)**

15.16 A 30-year-old man requests help for an opioid abuse disorder. He has used large quantities of prescription narcotics obtained on the streets and will also inject heroin when it is available. He has tried to quit these drugs on his own several times without success. Which of the following is the best option to treat his opioid use disorder and reduce his risk of relapse and criminal activity?

A. Referral to Narcotics Anonymous.
B. Detoxification with clonidine followed by outpatient counseling.
C. Referral to a methadone maintenance program.
D. Prescribing naltrexone.
E. Detoxification with clonidine followed by referral to an intensive outpatient program.

The correct response is option C: Referral to a methadone maintenance program.

Methadone maintenance programs have been shown to reduce risk of relapse, depression, criminal activity and to improve the functional status of patients with opioid use disorders. These programs typically provide counseling services in addition to the medication. Methadone maintenance programs have been shown to be better than abstinence in reducing relapse rates. The other response options (A, B, E) could each be useful, but option C is the most appropriate choice for this patient. Naltrexone (option D) has no role in the treatment of opioid use disorders. **(p. 418)**

15.17 A 26-year-old woman comes to your office seeking help for anxiety and panic attacks. She was last seen by your colleague a week ago, but she reports that she has lost her prescription for alprazolam. She asks you to write a new prescription for alprazolam 3 mg four times daily. She reports that nothing else works and that she has allergies to the selective serotonin reuptake inhibitors. Which of the following is *not* a valid reason to have serious concerns about prescribing alprazolam to this patient?

A. Concern about doctor-shopping behavior.
B. Report that "nothing else works."
C. Report of severe allergies to other medications commonly used to treat anxiety.
D. Report of a lost prescription.
E. Lethality of benzodiazepines in overdose.

The correct response is option E: Lethality of benzodiazepines in overdose.

Benzodiazepines have a very high therapeutic window and are not often lethal in overdose (option E). Options A–D all constitute very good reasons to have serious concerns about prescribing this patient a benzodiazepine. **(pp. 419–420)**

15.18 A 23-year-old man with no previous psychiatric history is brought to the emergency room by the police for agitated and disorganized behavior. He is paranoid and believes that the government is sending him messages through a microchip that was implanted in one of his teeth. He has not slept for 3 days. He is distractible in interview but otherwise oriented. A urine drug screen is positive for amphetamine. He is otherwise medically stable and is admitted to the psychiatry unit. What is the best course of treatment for this patient's psychotic symptoms?

A. Supportive care and possibly short-term use of antipsychotic.
B. Antipsychotic therapy for 6 months.
C. Cognitive-behavioral psychotherapy.
D. Imipramine.
E. Lithium.

The correct response is option A: Supportive care and possibly short-term use of antipsychotic.

Stimulant-induced psychoses generally resolve with sobriety; therefore, supportive care and a short-term antipsychotic is the best course of treatment (option A). Long-term use of an antipsychotic (option B) is not necessary. Antidepressants (option D) and psychotherapy (option C) will not treat the psychosis. The patient's insomnia and psychotic symptoms are more likely due to methamphetamine use than bipolar I disorder given the urine drug screen results, therefore use of lithium (option E) is not indicated. **(p. 424)**

15.19 What form of therapy for substance use disorders rewards patients for appropriate behavior (e.g., giving patients who submit clean urine samples vouchers that can be exchanged for retail goods and services)?

A. Contingency management.
B. Motivational interviewing.
C. Cognitive-behavioral therapy.
D. Behavioral activation.
E. Twelve-step program.

The correct response is option A: Contingency management.

Contingency management rewards appropriate behavior with material goods (option A). Motivational interviewing (option B) helps patients to make their own argument for change. Cognitive-behavioral therapy (option C) addresses negative automatic thoughts and core beliefs and explores how thoughts, feelings, and behaviors relate. Behavioral activation (option D) is a method that encourages depressed patients to reengage in their usual activities in spite of depression. Twelve-step programs (option E) such as Alcoholics Anonymous provide regular supportive community meetings to help patients maintain and achieve abstinence from alcohol and other substances of abuse. **(pp. 408, 427–428, 524 [Chapter 20])**

15.20 Which of the following treatments has a role in treating gambling disorder?

A. Gamblers Anonymous (GA).
B. Naltrexone.
C. Motivational interviewing.
D. Cognitive-behavioral therapy (CBT).
E. All of the above.

The correct response is option E: All of the above.

While there are no standard treatments for gambling disorder, each of the treatments listed has a role. GA is a self-help group patterned after Alcoholics Anonymous and provides support and encouragement to persons in recovery from gambling disorder. Naltrexone has been shown in clinical trials to reduce gambling urges. Motivational interviewing and CBT are often combined during the psychotherapeutic treatment of gambling disorder. **(pp. 428–431)**

CHAPTER 16

Neurocognitive Disorders

16.1 Which of the following is a diagnostic category (or categories) new to DSM-5 for the diagnosis of neurocognitive disorders?

A. Social cognitive disorder.
B. Major neurocognitive disorder.
C. Major cognitive impairment disorder.
D. Mild neurocognitive disorder.
E. Major neurocognitive and mild neurocognitive disorders.

The correct response is option E: Major neurocognitive and mild neurocognitive disorders.

DSM-5 has transformed the classification of the neurocognitive disorders by introducing two new categories—major neurocognitive disorder and mild neurocognitive disorder—that are distinguished on the basis of severity. Diagnostic criteria are provided for each followed by criteria for specific etiological subtypes (e.g., major neurocognitive disorder due to Alzheimer's disease). Mild neurocognitive disorder is an important new category because it acknowledges less severe levels of impairment that can also be a focus of care. **(p. 433)**

16.2 Processing speed is a part of which cognitive domain?

A. Social cognition.
B. Complex attention.
C. Learning and memory.
D. Executive function.
E. Language.

The correct response is option B: Complex attention.

The criteria for major and mild neurocognitive disorders are based on six defined key cognitive domains. They are complex attention, executive function (option D), learning and memory (option C), language (option E), perceptual motor ability, and social cognition (option A). Complex attention encompasses sustained attention, divided attention, selective attention, and processing speed (option B). **(pp. 434–435)**

16.3 Which of the following is *not* a risk factor for delirium?

A. Use of narcotics.
B. Recent surgery.
C. Older age.
D. Preexisting depression.
E. Systemic infection.

The correct response is option D: Preexisting depression.

Elderly patients are at high risk for delirium (option C), especially those older than 80 years. Additional risk factors include a preexisting dementia, recent surgery (option B), bone fractures, systemic infections (option E), and recent use of narcotics (option A) or antipsychotics. Pre-existing depression is not a known risk factor (option D). **(p. 436)**

16.4 Which of the following is *least* consistent with delirium?

A. Fluctuation in mental status throughout the day.
B. Disturbance of memory.
C. Occurrence in a hospitalized patient receiving high doses of narcotics.
D. Patient reports of visual and tactile hallucinations.
E. Insidious onset.

The correct response is option E: Insidious onset.

Delirium typically has an acute onset over a few days rather than an insidious onset over weeks to months (option E). Visual and tactile hallucinations (option D) are common in delirium, although they are not required for the diagnosis. High-dose narcotics (option

C) can induce delirium, although delirium is a syndrome that can develop through a wide variety of etiologies. Fluctuations in mental status throughout the day and memory disturbance (options A, B) are features of delirium. **(pp. 435–437)**

16.5 In which of the following patients with delirium is a benzodiazepine *least* likely to worsen delirium?

A. A highly agitated 25-year-old man hospitalized for 2 weeks for encephalopathy.
B. A calm 32-year-old woman hospitalized for 1 week for pneumonia.
C. A 65-year-old alcoholic man hospitalized for the past 3 days recovering from abdominal surgery.
D. An agitated 75-year-old woman with sepsis who reports vivid visual hallucinations.
E. Any patient with delirium.

The correct response is option C: A 65-year-old alcoholic man hospitalized for the past 3 days recovering from abdominal surgery.

A benzodiazepine may be helpful for the surgical patient with alcoholism because it is possible that this patient's delirium is due to alcohol withdrawal. One would want to make a thorough assessment before recommending benzodiazepines in this case. When alcohol withdrawal is not present, benzodiazepines should be avoided because they can worsen delirium. **(pp. 438–439)**

16.6 Which of the following would distinguish a major neurocognitive disorder from a mild neurocognitive disorder?

A. Decline in memory from baseline.
B. Presence of word finding difficulties.
C. Presence of impairment on neuropsychological assessment.
D. Acute onset over days.
E. Impairment in ability to live independently.

The correct response is option E: Impairment in ability to live independently.

Major neurocognitive disorder causes an impairment in a person's ability to live independently, whereas a mild neurocognitive disorder does not (option E). Acute onset over days is more characteristic of a delirium (option D). Both major and mild neurocognitive disorders show some degree of impairment on neuropsychological assessment (option C), but the degree of impairment will be greater for major neurocognitive disorders. Patients with either major or mild neurocognitive disorders can present with memory impairment (option A) or word finding difficulties (option B). **(pp. 439–441)**

16.7 What percentage of patients with Alzheimer's disease develop psychotic symptoms such as hallucinations and delusions as their illness progresses?

A. 1%.
B. 5%.
C. 10%.
D. 25%.
E. 50%.

The correct response is option E: 50%.

About half of patients with Alzheimer's disease develop hallucinations and delusions. **(p. 442)**

16.8 A 67-year-old retired accountant presents to his family physician accompanied by his wife. His wife reports that he has been having progressive difficulty remembering appointments and important dates over the past 2 years, and she no longer allows him to drive. There are no current safety concerns at home. Brief cognitive assessment shows that he has impairment in short-term recall and has difficulty drawing a clock. What is the next best step in management of this case?

A. Referral to a skilled nursing facility.
B. Medical workup.
C. Neuropsychological assessment.
D. Start donepezil.
E. Referral to a psychiatrist to confirm diagnosis of neurocognitive disorder.

The correct response is option B: Medical workup.

All patients with a suspected neurocognitive disorder should have a medical workup to look for potential reversible causes of neurocognitive disorder. Suggested studies are a complete blood count; liver, thyroid, and renal function tests; serologic tests for syphilis and HIV; urinalysis; electrocardiogram; and chest X ray. Serum electrolytes, serum glucose, and vitamin B_{12} and folate levels should be measured. Brain imaging should be obtained; an electroencephalogram may be helpful as well if there is a concern for seizure activity. **(pp. 444–445)**

16.9 Which test can distinguish Alzheimer's disease from other neurocognitive disorders?

A. Magnetic resonance imaging (MRI).
B. Functional MRI.
C. Fluorodeoxyglucose positron emission tomography (PET) scan.
D. Lumbar puncture.
E. Alzheimer's disease can only be confirmed on autopsy.

The correct response is option C: Fluorodeoxyglucose positron emission tomography (PET) scan.

Fluorodeoxyglucose PET imaging can distinguish Alzheimer's disease from other neurocognitive disorders. It will show characteristic parietal and temporal hypometabolism. Options A, B, and D may be useful in a medical workup of dementia. An autopsy (option E) is the definitive test for Alzheimer's, but not in the living patient! **(p. 444)**

16.10 A 59-year-old woman is brought to her family physician accompanied by her spouse. She has had worsening of short-term memory and progressive apathy over the past month. She also reports low mood, insomnia, and low appetite, and she has lost 10 lbs. since the symptoms begin. She answers "I don't know" to many basic questions on a brief cognitive assessment. Which of the following medications would be of most benefit to this patient?

A. Donepezil.
B. Tacrine.
C. Sertraline.

D. Aripiprazole.

E. Memantine.

The correct response is option C: Sertraline.

In addition to memory disturbance, this patient endorses symptoms consistent with a major depressive episode. This is called *pseudodementia,* but it is not a DSM-5 diagnosis. In these cases, an antidepressant such as sertraline will treat the depression thereby improving cognition. However, the person with a pseudodementia is at risk for developing a neurocognitive disorder in the future. **(p. 446)**

16.11 Which of the following is most specific for Alzheimer's disease?

A. Neurofibrillary tangles.

B. β-Amyloid plaques.

C. Hyperphosphorylated tau protein.

D. Apolipoprotein E polymorphism.

E. All of the above are equally specific changes.

The correct response is option B: β-Amyloid plaques.

β-Amyloid plaques in the brain are a characteristic histopathological change in Alzheimer's disease (option B). Neurofibrillary tangles (option A), which are made up of hyperphosphorylated tau proteins (option C), are found in other neurodegenerative diseases in addition to patients with Alzheimer's disease. Apolipoprotein E polymorphisms (option D) influence an individual's risk of developing Alzheimer's disease. **(p. 449)**

16.12 Primary progressive aphasia and a behavioral-variant subtype occur in which neurocognitive disorder?

A. Alzheimer's disease.

B. Frontotemporal neurocognitive disorder.

C. Neurocognitive disorder with Lewy bodies.

D. Vascular neurocognitive disorder.

E. None of the above.

The correct response is option B: Frontotemporal neurocognitive disorder.

Frontotemporal dementia includes a behavioral variant and three language subtypes that present with progressive aphasia. **(p. 450)**

16.13 Which neurocognitive disorder is sometimes associated with rapid eye movement (REM) sleep behavior disorder?

A. Alzheimer's disease.
B. Frontotemporal neurocognitive disorder.
C. Neurocognitive disorder with Lewy bodies.
D. Vascular neurocognitive disorder.
E. None of the above.

The correct response is option C: Neurocognitive disorder with Lewy bodies.

Neurocognitive disorder with Lewy bodies is associated with REM sleep behavior disorder. **(p. 450)**

16.14 A 67-year-old man is brought in to see his family physician by his family. They are concerned because he has had progressive difficulty keeping up with daily chores at home and is more irritable than usual. He tells the physician that he wouldn't be so irritable if his wife hadn't moved so many of her friends into the house. His wife reports that they live alone, and he seems to see people who aren't there. The patient is oriented and attends to the interview without difficulty. The physician notices that the patient has a shuffling gait. What is the most likely diagnosis?

A. Alzheimer's disease.
B. Frontotemporal neurocognitive disorder.
C. Neurocognitive disorder with Lewy bodies.
D. Vascular neurocognitive disorder.
E. Dementia.

The correct response is option C: Neurocognitive disorder with Lewy bodies.

Neurocognitive disorder with Lewy bodies is associated with visual hallucinations. The first cognitive changes noted tend to be problems with executive function, complex attention, and subtle personality changes (option C). Hallucinations can occur in other neurocognitive disorders such as Alzheimer's disease (option A), but they usually occur later in the disease process. Parkinsonian features may begin after the onset of cognitive decline. A person with frontotemporal neurocognitive disorder (option B) is likely to present with apathy or disinhibition. Vascular neurocognitive disorder (option D) is common, but a person with this disorder is likely to present with focal neurological deficits. Dementia (option E) is a generic term that in DSM-5 has been replaced by the term *neurocognitive disorder*. **(p. 450)**

16.15 A rapid, progressive stepwise cognitive decline suggests which neurocognitive disorder?

A. Alzheimer's disease.
B. Frontotemporal neurocognitive disorder.
C. Neurocognitive disorder with Lewy bodies.
D. Vascular neurocognitive disorder.
E. Delirium.

The correct response is option D: Vascular neurocognitive disorder.

Vascular neurocognitive disorder will often show a stepwise decline, because the cognitive deficits are secondary to ischemic events (option D). Delirium (option E) has an acute onset of impairment in attention and altered sensorium, and it is often reversible with treatment of the underlying cause. Alzheimer's disease, frontotemporal neurocognitive disorder, and neurocognitive disorder with Lewy bodies (options A–C) present with an insidious, gradual decline rather than stepwise decline. **(pp. 448, 450–451)**

16.16 A 25-year-old man recently diagnosed with an HIV infection sees his internist to address some concerns. He has read about "HIV dementia," and he asks his physician about his risk of developing this complication. What is the most accurate response?

A. It's a rare complication, so your risk is low.
B. You have a high risk of developing this condition at some point.
C. We can't determine this at the present.
D. There's a fair chance you may eventually develop some mild cognitive problems, but your risk of developing severe cognitive problems is low.
E. None of the above.

The correct response is option D: There's a fair chance you may eventually develop some mild cognitive problems, but your risk of developing severe cognitive problems is low.

Up to 25% of patients with HIV will develop a mild neurocognitive disorder, but the chances of developing a major neurocognitive disorder secondary to HIV are less than 5%. **(p. 453)**

16.17 Which of the following findings is characteristic of Creutzfeldt-Jakob disease?

A. Triphasic complexes on electroencephalogram (EEG).
B. Diffuse slowing on EEG.
C. Hypocretin deficiency.
D. Degeneration of the mammillary bodies.
E. Hypometabolism of parietal and temporal areas on PET scan.

The correct response is option A: Triphasic complexes on EEG.

Triphasic complexes on EEG are characteristic of Creutzfeldt-Jakob disease (option A), although a new variant that lacks this finding has been identified. Diffuse slowing on EEG (option B) suggests delirium. Hypocretin deficiency (option C) suggests the sleep disorder narcolepsy. Degeneration of the mammillary bodies (option D) occurs in Wernicke-Korsakoff syndrome. Hypometabolism of parietal and temporal areas on PET scan (option E) is characteristic of Alzheimer's disease. **(pp. 402 [Chapter 15], 438, 444, 453–454)**

16.18 Dementia, gait disturbance, and urinary incontinence are the classic triad of which medical condition that can cause a neurocognitive disorder?

A. Pellagra.
B. Prion disease.
C. Subdural hematoma.
D. Alcohol use.
E. Normal pressure hydrocephalus.

The correct response is option E: Normal pressure hydrocephalus.

Normal pressure hydrocephalus is classically associated with cognitive decline, gait disturbance, and urinary incontinence (option E). Long-term, heavy alcohol use (option D) can cause some cognitive decline and some cerebellar degeneration, which may result in some degree of ataxia. Subdural hematoma (option C) and pellagra (option A) can cause cognitive disorder, but the forms that these cognitive disorders take do not have established characteristic features. Prion disease (option B) causes a rapidly progressive, fatal cognitive decline that is associated with myoclonus and akinetic mutism. (pp. 454–456)

16.19 Which of the following medications is an appropriate choice to help with nighttime agitation, or "sundowning," in patients with neurocognitive disorders?

A. Lithium.
B. Carbamazepine.
C. Divalproex.
D. Trazodone.
E. Chlorpromazine.

The correct response is option D: Trazodone.

A bedtime dose of trazodone can help with sundowning in patients with neurocognitive disorders (option D). Chlorpromazine (option E) and other low-potency, first-generation antipsychotics should be avoided because their anticholinergic side effects can worsen cognition. Lithium, carbamazepine, and divalproex (options A–C) have no clear role in treating the behavioral complications of neurocognitive disorders. (p. 458)

16.20 Which of the following cognitive-enhancing drugs works on N-methyl-D-aspartate (NMDA) receptors?

A. Donepezil.
B. Tacrine.
C. Memantine.
D. Rivastigmine.
E. Galantamine.

The correct response is option C: Memantine.

Memantine blocks NMDA receptors that normally bind glutamate (option C). The agents in options A, B, D, and E are cholinesterase inhibitors. **(p. 457)**

16.21 Why has the U.S. Food and Drug Administration (FDA) issued a black box warning about the use of second-generation antipsychotics in elderly patients with neurocognitive disorders?

A. They are associated with an increased rate of cognitive decline.
B. They are associated with severe gastrointestinal side effects.
C. They are associated with an increased risk of mortality.
D. Liver enzymes must be monitored regularly.
E. They have no benefit for managing disruptive behaviors in patients with neurocognitive disorders.

The correct response is option C: They are associated with an increased risk of mortality.

The FDA issued a warning about the use of second-generation antipsychotics in elderly patients with neurocognitive disorders because of an increased risk of mortality (option C). These agents can help control disruptive behaviors and psychosis (option E). While these drugs can cause gastrointestinal symptoms, the symptoms are usually not severe and are not subject to a black box warning (option D). Liver enzymes must be monitored with use of the cholinesterase inhibitor tacrine (option D), which is not in common use. There is no evidence that second-generation antipsychotics are associated with cognitive decline (option A). **(pp. 458–459)**

— CHAPTER 17 —

Personality Disorders

17.1   Which was the first DSM to include disturbances of personality?

A. DSM-I.
B. DSM-II.
C. DSM-III.
D. DSM-IV.
E. DSM-5.

The correct response is option A: DSM-I.

DSM-I included seven types of personality disturbance, and personality disorders have been a part of each subsequent DSM. The disorders are unchanged from DSM-IV to DSM-5. **(p. 461)**

17.2   Which of the following is *not* true of the general criteria of a personality disorder?

A. The behavior is consistent with the individual's cultural expectations.
B. It is stable over time, with onset in adolescence or early adulthood.
C. The disorder leads to distress or impairment.
D. The disorder is not limited to episodes of illness.
E. All of the above are part of the general criteria of a personality disorder.

The correct response is option A: The behavior is consistent with the individual's cultural expectations.

271

Personality disorders represent an enduring pattern of inner experience and behavior that deviates markedly from the expectations of an individual's culture (option A). Options B, C, and D are part of the general criteria of a personality disorder. **(p. 462)**

17.3 A patient has long-standing discrete episodes of mania and depression dating to late adolescence. During manic episodes, he displays elevated mood, decreased sleep, pressured speech, and flight of ideas. The episodes typically result in psychiatric hospitalization. During the manic episodes, he engages in antisocial behavior, including committing assaults and writing bad checks. He is a quiet, law-abiding citizen between episodes of mania. What is the best diagnosis?

A. Antisocial personality disorder.
B. Bipolar I disorder.
C. Personality disorder due to bipolar disorder.
D. Bipolar I disorder plus antisocial personality disorder.
E. None of the above.

The correct response is option B: Bipolar I disorder.

This patient cannot be diagnosed with antisocial personality disorder (option A) because his antisocial behavior is limited to episodes of mania. For that reason, bipolar I disorder plus antisocial personality disorder (option D) is also inappropriate. Per the general criteria of a personality disorder, deviant behavior cannot be limited to discrete episodes of illness. Personality disorder secondary to bipolar disorder (option C) is not a DSM-5 diagnosis. **(pp. 461–463, 475–477)**

17.4 A patient has long-standing discrete episodes of mania and depression dating back to late adolescence. During the manic episodes, he has elevated mood, decreased sleep, pressured speech, and flight of ideas that typically result in psychiatric hospitalization. He gets into more legal trouble than usual during these periods, but even during periods of euthymia, he tends to engage in illegal activities such as shoplifting and burglary. He has done so since early adolescence, and he does not show any remorse for these actions. How would you best diagnose this patient?

A. Antisocial personality disorder.
B. Bipolar I disorder.

C. Personality disorder due to bipolar disorder.

D. Bipolar affective disorder type 1 plus antisocial personality disorder.

E. None of the above.

The correct response is option D: Bipolar affective disorder type 1 plus antisocial personality disorder.

In contrast to the patient in question 17.3, this patient has a long-standing pattern of antisocial behavior that is not limited to episodes of his illness. Therefore, it is most appropriate to diagnose him with both antisocial personality disorder and bipolar affective disorder (option D). Personality disorder secondary to bipolar disorder (option C) is not a valid diagnosis. Bipolar I disorder and antisocial personality disorder (options A, B) are inappropriate because they do not account for the combination of disorders seen in this man. **(pp. 462–463, 465, 474–477)**

17.5   Which of the following does *not* represent a major personality trait according to personality theorists who favor a dimensional perspective?

A. Extraversion.

B. Agreeableness.

C. Openness to experience.

D. Genuineness.

E. Neuroticism.

The correct response is option D: Genuineness.

The best-known dimensional personality model was developed by psychologists Paul Costa and Robert McCrae and is known as the five-factor model. The traits outlined by the model include extraversion, agreeableness (options A, B), conscientiousness (not genuineness [option D]), openness to experience, and neuroticism (options C, E). **(p. 463)**

17.6   Which personality disorder is more common in men than in women?

A. Antisocial personality disorder.

B. Borderline personality disorder.

C. Histrionic personality disorder.

D. Dependent personality disorder.

E. Schizotypal personality disorder.

The correct response is option A: Antisocial personality disorder.

Antisocial personality disorder is more common in men (option A). Borderline, histrionic, and dependent personality disorders (options B–D) are more common in women. Schizotypal personality disorder (option E) is equally common in men and women. **(p. 464)**

17.7   Which is the only personality disorder with an age requirement and a requirement that certain childhood behaviors have continuity with adult traits?

A. Antisocial personality disorder.

B. Borderline personality disorder.

C. Avoidant personality disorder.

D. Dependent personality disorder.

E. Schizotypal personality disorder.

The correct response is option A: Antisocial personality disorder.

Antisocial personality disorder cannot be diagnosed before age 18 years, and the diagnosis requires evidence of a childhood conduct disorder (option A). DSM-5 requires that the maladaptive personality features be present for at least 1 year if a personality disorder is diagnosed at an age less than 18 years. The other personality disorders (e.g., options B–E) do not have an age requirement. Although no other personality disorder has child or adolescent criteria, research suggests that behavioral precursors such as affective lability or impulsivity can sometimes be traced back to childhood. Furthermore, personality pathology in childhood or adolescence is predictive of adult maladjustment and the development of a personality disorder. **(p. 464)**

17.8   Does the diagnosis of a personality disorder tend to be stable over time?

A. Most personality disorders are diagnostically stable throughout life, but the severity may diminish with age.

B. Most personality disorders are diagnostically stable, and symptoms severity is stable.

C. Severity of personality disorders diminishes, and many people will make a full psychosocial recovery.
D. Severity of the personality disorder diminishes, but many people will still have some degree of interpersonal dysfunction.
E. None of the above.

The correct response is option D: Severity of the personality disorder diminishes, but many people will still have some degree of interpersonal dysfunction.

The severity of personality disorders tends to decrease as patients age, and many patients diagnosed with a personality disorder will no longer meet full criteria for a given disorder with time. Most will continue to have some degree of impairment in important life domains. **(pp. 464–465)**

17.9   Which of the following has *not* been shown to contribute to the risk of developing a personality disorder?

A. Being a victim of child abuse.
B. Witnessing domestic violence in the home.
C. Parental divorce or separation.
D. Parental absence.
E. Arrested psychosexual development.

The correct response is option E: Arrested psychosexual development.

Psychoanalysts have postulated that maladaptive personality traits arise from arrested psychosexual development (option E), but there is no evidence to support this view. Options A–D have all been shown to contribute to the risk of developing a personality disorder. **(pp. 466–467)**

17.10 Which personality disorder is associated with impaired smooth pursuit eye movement, impaired performance on tests of executive function, and increased ventricular-brain ratio on computed tomography?

A. Antisocial personality disorder.
B. Borderline personality disorder.
C. Schizotypal personality disorder.

D. Schizoid personality disorder.

E. Avoidant personality disorder.

The correct response is option C: Schizotypal personality disorder.

Schizotypal personality disorder, long considered to fall within the spectrum of disorders related to schizophrenia, is associated with impaired smooth pursuit eye movement, impaired performance on tests of executive function, and increased ventricular-brain ratio on computed tomography. **(p. 466)**

17.11 Which personality disorder is associated with low resting pulse, low skin conductance, and increased amplitude on event-related potentials?

A. Antisocial personality disorder.

B. Borderline personality disorder.

C. Schizotypal personality disorder.

D. Schizoid personality disorder.

E. Avoidant personality disorder.

The correct response is option A: Antisocial personality disorder.

Antisocial personality disorder is associated with low resting pulse, low skin conductance, and increased amplitude on event-related potentials. These findings suggest to some that antisocial persons are chronically underaroused and seek out potentially risky situations to raise their arousal to more optimal levels. **(p. 466)**

17.12 A 27-year-old software engineer seeks psychiatric treatment for anxiety. He has lived alone all of his adult life. Outside of work, he has no social contacts apart from a weekly phone call to his mother. He spends most of his free time playing video games, and he expresses little interest in developing more social relationships or having a romantic relationship. He does not endorse any symptoms of major depression or psychosis. He is very stiff and formal in interview and displays little emotion. What is the best diagnosis?

A. Avoidant personality disorder.

B. Schizotypal personality disorder.

C. Schizoid personality disorder.

D. Autism spectrum disorder.

E. Antisocial personality disorder.

The correct response is option C: Schizoid personality disorder.

Patients with schizoid personality disorder have a profound defect in the ability to form personal relationships and to respond to others in a meaningful way (option C). Patients with avoidant personality disorder (option A) typically desire social contact, but their anxiety interferes with developing relationships in the absence of significant reassurance. Patients with schizotypal personality disorder (option B) tend to have few relationships but are odd and eccentric with unusual thinking and speech. Although autism spectrum disorder (option D) is not a bad choice in that people with these disorders often have few relationships, they also have significant impairments in social communication and restricted and repetitive patterns of behavior, which the patient in the vignette does not have. Patients with antisocial personality disorder (option E) are antisocial in the sense that they do not have respect for the rights of others not because of impaired social skills. **(pp. 101–103 [Chapter 4], 471–475, 483)**

17.13 You see a 33-year-old unemployed man in the outpatient clinic. He reports that he would like your assistance in getting disability for "anxiety." He says that for as long as he recalls, he has felt uncomfortable in social situations because he fears that other people will not understand him. He has never married and has no children. He has trouble maintaining employment due to anxiety. He sometimes thinks that magazine articles have special messages for him and may see shadows that look like people or animals. He has been trying to learn how to communicate telepathically by studying a "new age" book purchased on the Internet but has not been successful. He denies any history of auditory hallucinations and does not appear to have delusions. What is the best diagnosis?

A. Schizophrenia.

B. Schizotypal personality disorder.

C. Avoidant personality disorder.

D. Schizoid personality disorder.

E. Schizoaffective disorder.

The correct response is option B: Schizotypal personality disorder.

The man in the vignette best meets the spirit of schizotypal personality disorder (option B). Such patients are odd and eccentric and typically have unusual thinking and speech. Patients with paranoid personality disorder are distrustful of others but otherwise are not especially odd. Patients with schizoid personality disorder (option D) have a profound defect in the ability to form personal relationships and to respond to others in a meaningful way, but also tend not to be otherwise strange or eccentric. Patients with schizophrenia or schizoaffective disorder (options A, E) have frank delusions and hallucinations, in contrast to the nonpsychotic symptoms of patients with schizotypal personality disorder. Patients with avoidant personality disorder (option C) have difficulty forming relationships due to severe social anxiety. (pp. 471–473)

17.14 Which of the following is *not* a trait of histrionic personality disorder?

A. Unease in situations in which one is not the center of attention.
B. Inappropriate sexually seductive or provocative behavior.
C. Rapidly shifting and shallow expression of emotions.
D. Transient, stress-related paranoid ideation or severe dissociative symptoms.
E. Self-dramatization, theatricality, and exaggerated expression of emotion.

The correct response is option D: Transient, stress-related paranoid ideation or severe dissociative symptoms.

Transient, stress-related paranoid ideation or severe dissociative symptoms is a trait of borderline personality disorder (option D). Options A–C and E represent traits of histrionic personality disorder. (pp. 477–480)

17.15 A 26-year-old woman comes to your clinic to establish care for her mood swings that other psychiatrists have diagnosed as "bipolar disorder." She has persistent depression and severe mood swings, but she has never had a period of decreased sleep, pressured speech, or disinhibition that lasted for several days. She uses a razor blade to make small cuts on her forearms when anxious or upset but denies that she does this to kill herself. She has had several psychiatric hospitalizations for suicidal ideation, and she has overdosed multiple times. She endorses a deep fear that her loved ones will abandon her, and she has chronic feelings of emptiness. After your interview, she says that she thinks you are the best doctor she has ever had and that she has great confidence in your abilities. She speaks very poorly of her previous psychiatrist. What is the most likely diagnosis?

A. Bipolar II disorder.
B. Histrionic personality disorder.
C. Borderline personality disorder.
D. Dependent personality disorder.
E. Schizotypal personality disorder.

The correct response is option C: Borderline personality disorder.

Patients with borderline personality disorder suffer from mood and interpersonal instability and often have fears of abandonment (option C). Patients with bipolar disorder (option A) have discrete episodes of mania and depression. Histrionic personality disorder (option B) is characterized by attention-seeking behavior and shallow affect but not self-harm or mood instability. Patients with dependent personality disorder (option D) are overly reliant on others to meet their needs. Patients with schizotypal personality disorder (option E) have odd speech and thinking but do not report mood instability and are not chronically suicidal. **(pp. 161 [Chapter 6], 473, 477, 480–482, 484–485)**

17.16 A 40-year-old business executive seeks treatment for depression. She reports being upset since a colleague was given a promotion that she feels was rightfully hers. Her long-term goal is to become the CEO of a major global corporation. During the session, she questions the therapist's credentials, and at one point she accuses the therapist of being envious of her superior social status. She does not return after the first session and later tells an acquaintance that it was because the therapist didn't give her the admiration that she deserves. What is the most likely diagnosis?

A. Antisocial personality disorder.
B. Borderline personality disorder.
C. Narcissistic personality disorder.

D. Dependent personality disorder.

E. Histrionic personality disorder.

The correct response is option C: Narcissistic personality disorder.

Narcissistic personality disorder is characterized by exaggerated sense of self-importance and lack of empathy (option C). The other response options are not plausible, although many narcissistic persons will have symptoms consistent with some of the other personality disorders. Patients with dependent personality disorder (option D) are overly reliant on others to meet their needs. Histrionic personality disorder (option E) is characterized by attention-seeking behavior and shallow affect. Patients with borderline personality disorder (option B) have mood and interpersonal instability and deep fears of abandonment. Patients with antisocial personality disorder (option A) habitually violate the rights of others. (pp. 474–475, 477, 479–481, 484–485)

17.17 Which of the following does *not* represent a recommended treatment for borderline personality disorder?

A. Dialectical behavior therapy.

B. Benzodiazepine tranquilizers for accompanying anxiety.

C. Systems Training for Emotional Predictability and Problem Solving (STEPPS).

D. Antipsychotic medications for accompanying perceptual distortions and anger dyscontrol.

E. Selective serotonin reuptake inhibitors (SSRIs) for depression.

The correct response is option B: Benzodiazepine tranquilizers for accompanying anxiety.

Although the treatment of patients with borderline personality disorder is challenging, many treatment options have been developed. There are now many psychotherapeutic programs that are evidence-based, including dialectical behavior therapy (option A) and STEPPS (option C). Although no medications are U.S. Food and Drug Administration (FDA) approved to treat any personality disorder, including borderline personality disorder, research show that depressed patients may benefit from antidepressants such as SSRIs (option E), whereas many symptoms of borderline personality disorder may improve with antipsychotic medications (option D). Benzodiazepines (option B) should be avoided in these patients because of their abuse potential and tendency to cause behavioral disinhibition. **(p. 479)**

17.18 Which of the following personality disorders is *not* a cluster C personality disorder?

A. Avoidant personality disorder.
B. Obsessive-compulsive personality disorder.
C. Histrionic personality disorder.
D. Dependent personality disorder.
E. All of the above are cluster C personality disorders.

The correct response is option C: Histrionic personality disorder.

The cluster C personality disorders are avoidant, obsessive-compulsive, and dependent personality disorders (options A, B, D). Histrionic personality disorder (option C) is a cluster B personality disorder. **(Table 17–1 [DSM-5 personality disorders], p. 462)**

17.19 Avoidant personality disorder can be very difficult to distinguish from which of the following disorders?

A. Social anxiety disorder.
B. Generalized anxiety disorder.
C. Panic disorder.
D. Persistent depressive disorder.
E. Autism spectrum disorder.

The correct response is option A: Social anxiety disorder.

Avoidant personality disorder symptoms overlap significantly with social anxiety disorder (option A). Several response options are plausible, but incorrect. Generalized anxiety disorder (option B) is accompanied by chronic anxiety but not interpersonal deficits. Panic disorder (option C) causes discrete episodes on anxious and panicky feelings but is not accompanied by social deficits, although it is often comorbid with social anxiety disorder. Persistent depressive disorder (option D) is characterized by chronic depression, and that may be accompanied by low self-esteem that can contribute to social withdrawal. Persons with autism spectrum disorder (option E) may be socially withdrawn and also have social communication deficits and restrictive, repetitive patterns of behavior. (pp. 483–484)

17.20   Ebenezer Scrooge comes to your practice seeking therapy for life dissatisfaction. He spends all of his time working even though he is very wealthy, and he is very reluctant to spend his money on basic amenities such as heating during the cold winter months. He engages in very little recreation and has very little social interaction, and he rejects his nephew's dinner invitations. He expresses rigid, controversial opinions, such as that donating to charity is wasteful given that his hard-earned tax dollars finance work houses and debtors' prisons. He micromanages his sole employee, but he reserves several tasks for himself for fear that his employee is not competent to handle these necessities to his satisfaction. What is the best diagnosis for this patient?

A. Schizoid personality disorder.
B. Narcissistic personality disorder.
C. Obsessive-compulsive personality disorder.
D. Avoidant personality disorder.
E. Antisocial personality disorder.

The correct response is option C: Obsessive-compulsive personality disorder.

Charles Dickens was a remarkable observer of human behavior and foibles, and he captures the essence of obsessive-compulsive personality disorder in his memorable character Ebenezer Scrooge (option C). The disorder is characterized by uncompromising rigidity and perfectionism to the exclusion of pleasurable activities. Scrooge may have some elements of narcissistic and antisocial personality disorders (options B, E) in that he appears to lack empathy for others such as his long-suffering assistant, Bob Cratchit. Schizoid personality disorder (option A) could be a plausible response, because Scrooge is emotionally cold and detached, but earlier in life, as Dickens reveals, he had a rich social life and enjoyed close relationships. There is no reason to believe he has an avoidant personality disorder (option D), because while he has a constricted social life, he does not appear to have feelings of inadequacy or interpersonal hypersensitivity. (pp. 486–487)

CHAPTER 18

Psychiatric Emergencies

18.1   Aggressive behavior is associated with which of the following findings in the cerebrospinal fluid (CSF)?

A. Dopamine excess.
B. Norepinephrine excess.
C. Serotonin deficiency.
D. Acetylcholine deficiency.
E. Glutamine excess.

The correct response is option C: Serotonin deficiency.

At a neurophysiological level, aggressive behavior has been associated with disturbed central nervous system serotonin function. Low CSF 5-hydroxyindoleacetic acid (5-HIAA) levels are correlated with impulsive violence, one of the best-replicated laboratory findings in psychiatry. (5-HIAA is a metabolite of serotonin.) It has been hypothesized that serotonin acts as the central nervous system's natural policing mechanism, helping to keep impulsive and violent behavior in check. **(p. 493)**

18.2   Which of the following is the single best predictor of future violent behavior?

A. Threats of violence.
B. Diagnosis of a severe mental illness (e.g., schizophrenia, bipolar disorder).
C. Prior psychiatric hospitalization.
D. Substance abuse history.
E. History of violence.

The correct response is option E: History of violence.

Although long-range predictions of violent behavior are beyond the skills of mental health professionals, they are in a position to predict violence in clinical settings. A patient's history of violent behavior is probably the single best predictor of future dangerousness (option E). Clinical wisdom suggests that past behavior predicts future behavior. The accuracy of predictions is improved in clinical populations that have high base rates for violence, such as patients on locked psychiatric inpatient units. That said, the importance of options A–D should not be dismissed in making a clinical assessment as well as, for example, inability to control anger, a history of impulsive behavior, paranoid ideation or frank psychosis. **(pp. 491–492; Table 18–1 [Clinical variables associated with violence], p. 495)**

18.3   Which of the following personality disorders is most associated with violent behavior?

A. Paranoid personality disorder.
B. Antisocial personality disorder.
C. Schizotypal personality disorder.
D. Narcissistic personality disorder.
E. Schizoid personality disorder.

The correct response is option B: Antisocial personality disorder.

Acting-out personality disorders such as antisocial and borderline personality disorders are associated with violent behavior, a fact that is reflected by their high prevalence among incarcerated persons. **(p. 493)**

18.4   Which of the following best describes the natural history of antisocial and borderline personality disorders?

A. Patients tend to act out more as they grow older.
B. Patients tend to act out less as they grow older.
C. Patients' tendency to act out does not change.
D. Patients only tend to act out less with age if they do not have a childhood history of conduct disorder.
E. Patients only tend to act out less with age if they do not have a childhood history of fire setting or cruelty to animals.

The correct response is option B: Patients tend to act out less as they grow older.

Acting-out behavior tends to change with advancing age (option C). With advancing age and maturity, patients with antisocial and borderline personality disorders tend to act out less (option B), not more (option A). Childhood history of conduct disorder is necessary to make the diagnosis of antisocial personality disorder (option D). A childhood history of fire setting and cruelty to animals increases risk of acting-out behavior in adulthood, but there is no reason to believe that their absence will nullify the tendency for acting out behaviors to diminish with age (option E). **(p. 493)**

18.5 A psychiatrist is called to evaluate a patient in the emergency room whose chief complaint is homicidal ideation. The psychiatrist remains calm and speaks softly. She seats herself for the interview and allows distance between her and the patient. She is careful to always make direct eye contact and to project empathy and concern. She asks nonjudgmental questions during the interview. Which of the following behaviors displayed by the psychiatrist is *not* recommended?

A. Speaking softly.
B. Sitting during the interview, because psychiatrists should stand in order to be ready to escape.
C. Projecting empathy and concern because it can seem patronizing to a violent patient.
D. Use of direct eye contact.
E. Asking nonjudgmental questions.

The correct response is option D: Use of direct eye contact.

Direct eye contact should be avoided when assessing potentially violent patients (option D). The clinician should speak softly, remain seated, project empathy and concern, and ask nonjudgmental questions (options A–C, E). **(p. 494)**

18.6 You are seeing a patient with schizophrenia in the emergency room. The patient acknowledges his diagnosis and reports a worsening of symptoms. He reports he has been hearing voices that have been telling him to kill a family member, something that he does not want to do. He has been hospitalized multiple times but does not have a history of violence. The patient is pleasant and cooperative. Which of the following is the most concerning risk factor for violence?

A. Lack of insight.
B. Stated desire to hurt or kill.
C. Presence of command hallucinations.
D. Diagnosis of schizophrenia.
E. History of psychiatric hospitalization.

The correct response is option C: Presence of command hallucinations.

The major risk factor for violence in this case is the presence of command hallucinations (option C). The patient shows some insight (option A) into his illness and does not voice a personal desire to follow through with this command (option B). Diagnosis of schizophrenia and history of psychiatric hospitalization (options D, E) are not in themselves major clinical variables associated with violence. **(Table 18–1 [Clinical variables associated with violence], p. 495)**

18.7 Which of the following combinations of medications is commonly given to calm acutely agitated patients?

A. Alprazolam and diphenhydramine.
B. Chlorpromazine and clonazepam.
C. Olanzapine and lorazepam.
D. Haloperidol and lorazepam.
E. Droperidol and alprazolam.

The correct response is option D: Haloperidol and lorazepam.

Haloperidol 2–5 mg and lorazepam 1–2 mg can be given to a patient every 30 minutes until sedation is achieved (option D). Many of the other medications are sedating, but the haloperidol-lorazepam combination has become standard practice for dealing with acute agitation. Droperidol is useful but is rarely used because of a black box warning (option E). **(p. 495)**

18.8 Fill in the blank: Suicide is the _____ leading cause of death in persons between ages 15 and 24 years.

A. First.
B. Second.
C. Third.
D. Fifth.
E. Eleventh.

The correct response is option C: Third.

Suicide is the third leading cause of death for persons between ages 15 and 24 years. It is the tenth most frequent cause of death for adults in general. **(p. 497)**

18.9   Which of the following is true with regard to most people who commit suicide?

A. They usually do not tell anyone before committing suicide.
B. They may tell a friend or family member but usually do not seek medical help.
C. They usually communicate their suicidal intentions to and see physicians before they die.
D. They usually see a physician but do not usually tell their physician that they are having suicidal thoughts.
E. They usually do not have a primary care physician.

The correct response is option C: They usually communicate their suicidal intentions to and see physicians before they die.

Most people who commit suicide communicate their suicidal intentions to and see physicians before they die. In fact, nearly two-thirds of suicidal persons communicate their suicidal intentions to others. Their communication may be as direct as reporting their plan and the date they intend to carry it out. Other communications are less obvious; for instance, a patient may say to his relatives, "You won't have to put up with me much longer." **(p. 497)**

18.10   Which individual probably is at highest risk of completing suicide?

A. 25-year-old, divorced African American man.
B. 55-year-old, married white woman.
C. 60-year-old, widowed white man.
D. 19-year-old, single African American woman.
E. 40-year-old, divorced white woman.

The correct response is option C: 60-year-old, widowed white man.

In the United States, most suicide completers tend to be older than 45 years, white, and separated, widowed, or divorced. **(p. 497)**

18.11 Which of the following is *not* associated with completed suicide?

A. Depressive disorder.
B. Male sex.
C. Hopelessness.
D. Substance use disorder.
E. African American race.

The correct response is option E: African American race.

Options A–D are all associated with elevated risk for completed suicide. African Americans have lower risk for suicide than whites (option E). **(p. 497; Figure 18–1 [Suicide rates in U.S. men and women by race and age: 2004], p. 498)**

18.12 Suicide is associated with which of the following in the CSF?

A. Dopamine excess.
B. Norepinephrine excess.
C. Serotonin deficiency.
D. Acetylcholine deficiency.
E. Glutamine excess.

The correct response is option C: Serotonin deficiency.

Low CSF levels of 5-HIAA, a serotonin metabolite, are correlated with both suicide and impulsive violence. **(pp. 499–500)**

18.13 What is the most common method used to commit suicide in the United States?

A. Overdose.
B. Cutting.
C. Hanging.
D. Firearm.
E. Jumping.

The correct response is option D: Firearm.

Firearms are the most common method used to commit suicide in the United States, perhaps because they are readily available and can be immediately lethal. Firearms are followed in frequency by poisoning (overdose), hanging, cutting, jumping, and other methods. **(p. 500)**

18.14 Which of the following is one of the strongest correlates of suicidal behavior, independent of psychiatric diagnosis?

A. Presence of a mental illness.
B. History of violence.
C. Recent psychiatric hospitalization.
D. Hopelessness.
E. Psychosocial stressors.

The correct response is option D: Hopelessness.

One of the strongest correlates of suicidal behavior is hopelessness, a finding independent of psychiatric diagnosis (option D). Most patients with mental illness do not ultimately commit suicide. Options A–C and E represent categories that are overly general. **(p. 500)**

18.15 For which group of patients is suicide frequently preceded by the loss of a relationship in the past year?

A. Alcoholic persons.
B. Patients with major depressive disorder.
C. Older patients with cognitive decline.
D. Adolescents with behavior problems.
E. People with a personality disorder.

The correct response is option A: Alcoholic persons.

More than 50% of alcoholic persons who commit suicide have a history of relationship loss—usually of an intimate relationship—within the year before suicide. **(p. 501)**

18.16 What medications are associated with lowered rates of suicide?

    A. Haloperidol.
    B. Lithium.
    C. Clozapine.
    D. Options A and B.
    E. Options B and C.

The correct response is option E: Options B and C.

Lithium has been reported to lower suicide risk in bipolar patients. Among the antipsychotics, only clozapine has been associated with lower rates of suicide. Neither other medications, electro-convulsive therapy, nor psychotherapy have been specifically shown to lower suicide risk. **(p. 504)**

─CHAPTER 19─

Legal Issues

19.1   Which of the following is a criminal and not a civil issue?

A. Determining whether to hospitalize a patient for acute homicidal ideation against his or her will.
B. Determining whether a patient with schizophrenia is capable of understanding court processes and assisting the court-appointed attorney.
C. Potential Health Insurance Portability and Accountability Act (HIPAA) violations.
D. Providing information about proposed treatments and alternatives and ensuring that the patient is capable of understanding these issues.
E. Determining whether a psychiatrist was negligent in his professional duties after abruptly terminating a doctor-patient relationship because the patient did not promptly pay a bill.

The correct response is option B: Determining whether a patient with schizophrenia is capable of understanding court processes and assisting the court-appointed attorney.

In the forensic world, the distinction between civil and criminal issues is fundamental. Whether a patient with schizophrenia is able to understand court processes and aid his or her attorney is an example of competence to stand trial, which is a criminal issue (option B). The other major criminal legal issue is determining criminal responsibility. Options A, C–E represent civil issues. **(p. 508)**

19.2   Which of the following is *not* a key criterion considered in civil commitment proceedings?

A. Mental illness.
B. Outpatient supports.
C. Dangerousness.
D. Disability.
E. Grave disability.

The correct response is option B: Outpatient supports.

The major criteria in determination of cases of civil commitment are mental illness, dangerousness, and disability (sometimes referred to as grave disability) (options A, C–E). Availability of outpatient supports is not one of the key criteria (option B), although it is an important consideration. **(p. 509)**

19.3   What level of evidence is generally required in cases of civil commitment?

A. Beyond a reasonable doubt.
B. Clear and convincing evidence.
C. Preponderance of the evidence.
D. Substantial evidence.
E. Some credible evidence.

The correct response is option B: Clear and convincing evidence.

The civil commitment process generally requires clear and convincing evidence (option B), a standard generally thought of as the level of proof needed for three of four reasonable people to agree. Options A, C–E represent other standards for evidence used in other legal proceedings. **(p. 510)**

19.4   Most states have provisions for

A. Involuntary inpatient treatment only.
B. Involuntary outpatient treatment only.
C. Both involuntary inpatient and outpatient treatment.
D. Neither involuntary nor voluntary outpatient treatment.
E. Voluntary outpatient treatment only.

The correct response is option C: Both involuntary inpatient and outpatient treatment.

Besides inpatient treatment, most states (44 of 50) have provisions for involuntary outpatient treatment. Such treatment may be used when the patient is not quite ill enough to merit inpatient care, but he or she presents some risk of harm to self or others because of mental illness and will not voluntarily comply with outpatient treatment. **(p. 511)**

19.5 In which of the following situations is it the *least* clear cut whether patient confidentiality may be broken according to our laws?

A. Reporting infectious disease such as tuberculosis or sexually transmitted infections.
B. Warning potential victims about threats made by patients.
C. Allowing access to medical charts for billing purposes.
D. Communicating with the family of a nonviolent psychiatric patient.
E. All of the above are clear cut cases in which confidentiality may be breached.

The correct response is option D: Communicating with the family of a nonviolent psychiatric patient.

In many instances, a psychiatrist may have good reason to want to have open communication with a patient's family because this may be in the best interest of the patient's care. However, it is not always legally clear cut whether the psychiatrist may break confidentiality in these cases (option D), although some states do have provisions to allow for this sort of communication. It is clear cut that confidentiality may be breached in regard to reporting of infectious diseases and warning potential victims about threats to their person (options A, B). Insurance companies, utilization review groups, and physician peer reviewers frequently have access to medical records for billing purposes (option C). **(pp. 511–512)**

19.6 What is the most common reason psychiatrists are sued for malpractice?

A. Failure to obtain informed consent.
B. Patient suicide.
C. Alleged injuries from psychotropic medications.
D. Patient abandonment.
E. Alleged electroconvulsive therapy–related injury.

The correct response is option B: Patient suicide.

It is important to know that psychiatrists are sued less frequently than other medical specialists. Nonetheless, patient suicide is the most common reason for a psychiatrist to be sued (option B). Options A and C–E are less common reasons for which a psychiatrist may be sued. **(pp. 513–514)**

19.7 What percentage of physicians will face at least one malpractice suit at some point in their careers?

A. 10%.
B. 35%.
C. 50%.
D. 65%.
E. 80%.

The correct response is option D: 65%.

Malpractice is negligence in the conduct of one's professional duties. The number of malpractice suits filed in the United States seems to climb each year. About two-thirds of physicians will experience at least one malpractice lawsuit during their professional career. The reaction among many physicians is to practice "defensive medicine," for example, ordering extra tests or refusing to treat certain patients. **(p. 513)**

19.8 According to the American Psychiatric Association, at what point does it become acceptable for a psychiatrist to have an intimate relationship with a former patient?

A. 6 months after termination of the doctor-patient relationship.
B. 1 year after termination of the doctor-patient relationship.
C. 3 years after termination of the doctor-patient relationship.
D. 10 years after termination of the doctor-patient relationship.
E. Never.

The correct response is option E: Never.

Sexual activity with current or former patients has become a well-publicized reason for malpractice litigation. Unlike errors in professional judgment, inappropriate sexual behavior with a patient is a voluntary act by a clinician and is therefore both preventable and excluded under most malpractice insurance policies. A psychiatrist may be expelled from professional associations, have his or her license suspended or revoked, and even face criminal charges for such "boundary violations." The American Psychiatric Association has made it clear that sexual contact with current or previous patients is inappropriate and unethical. **(p. 514)**

19.9   In order to be competent to stand trial, a defendant must meet all of the following criteria *except*

A. Being able to understand the nature of the charges against him or her.
B. Being able to understand the possible penalty.
C. Having been shown to have both bad behavior and blameworthy state of mind at the time of the offense.
D. Being able to understand the legal issues and procedures.
E. Being capable of working with an attorney in preparing the defense.

The correct response is option C: Having been shown to have both bad behavior and blameworthy state of mind at the time of the offense.

Competence to stand trial is a legal determination, not a medical one. It is determined by a judge according to national standards established by the U.S. Supreme Court in *Dusky v. United States*. To receive a fair trial, the following are required for establishing competence: a person must be able to understand the nature of the charges against him or her (option A), the possible penalty (option B), and the legal issues and procedures (option D), and he or she also must be able to work with the attorney in preparing the defense (option E). The presence of a mental illness, even a psychosis, generally does not render the defendant incompetent to stand trial. Competence to stand trial is assumed unless questioned by someone in the court. Bad behavior and blameworthy state of mind at the time of the offense (option C) are components of criminal responsibility rather than competence to stand trial. **(p. 515)**

19.10 According to current laws, a crime occurs when

A. Illegal behavior occurs, regardless of the perpetrator's state of mind.
B. Illegal behavior occurs and the perpetrator has a blameworthy state of mind.
C. A perpetrator has a blameworthy state of mind regardless of whether illegal behavior occurs.
D. Illegal behavior occurs and the person does not have demonstrable mental illness.
E. A person with mental illness has a blameworthy state of mind.

The correct response is option B: Illegal behavior occurs and the perpetrator has a blameworthy state of mind.

For a crime to occur, both bad behavior *(actus rea)* and a blameworthy state of mind *(mens rea)* must be present. A person may be so mentally ill as to lack this blameworthy state of mind by virtue of his or her disorder. In such a case, a person is said to lack criminal responsibility and is adjudicated as not guilty by reason of insanity. **(p. 515)**

19.11 Which of the following forms the basis of the insanity defense?

A. The *M'Naghten* standard.
B. The *Drummond* standard.
C. *Dusky v. United States.*
D. The *Tarasoff* rule.
E. The Peel Law.

The correct response is option A: The *M'Naghten* standard.

The *M'Naghten* standard established standards for determining criminal responsibility (option A). Drummond and Peel (options B, E) are names of individuals who were also involved in the M'Naghten case. The *Tarasoff* rule (option D) refers to the duty to protect. *Dusky v. United States* (option C) established standards for competency to stand trial rather than criminal responsibility. **(pp. 515–516)**

19.12 A patient reveals to his psychiatrist that he plans to harm a neighbor. The psychiatrist is obligated to break confidentiality in order to protect the potential victim. How shall the psychiatrist proceed?

A. Phone the neighbor to report the threat.
B. Phone the local police.
C. Ask the patient to phone the neighbor.
D. Report the threat to the local newspaper.
E. None of the above.

The correct response is option A: Phone the neighbor to report the threat.

The *Tarasoff* rule refers to the duty to protect third parties from the actions of patients in their care. On rare occasions, in the course of treating a patient, the patient may threaten to harm an identifiable third party. The psychiatrist has a legal responsibility to protect that third party and may break confidentiality by notifying the threatened person and/or the police. Although the approach to warning a third party has been debated, phoning the neighbor directly (option A) is the best option. Some psychiatrists will do this in the patient's presence. Phoning the local police (option B) may be worthwhile, but the message may not reach the intended victim. Asking the patient to phone the neighbor (option C) will probably not lead to the patient making the phone call. Reporting the threat to the local newspaper (option D) is not an acceptable response. **(pp. 515–516)**

19.13 A woman with a psychosis is charged with murder. During her pretrial screening, her speech is disorganized such that she cannot engage in coherent dialogue with her attorneys. Which of the following best describes her legal situation with regard to the charges against her?

A. She is competent to stand trial but not guilty by reason of insanity.
B. She is not competent to stand trial and also not guilty by reason of insanity.
C. She is not competent to stand trial, and whether she is not guilty by reason of insanity has yet to be demonstrated.
D. She is guilty but mentally ill.
E. She has diminished capacity.

The correct response is option C: She is not competent to stand trial, and whether she is not guilty by reason of insanity has yet to be demonstrated.

The ability to communicate with an attorney in order to prepare a defense is a component of competency to stand trial. Whether the patient has criminal responsibility has yet to be determined. Guilty but mentally ill and diminished capacity refer to degrees of criminal responsibility implemented by some states. **(p. 516)**

CHAPTER 20

Behavioral, Cognitive, and Psychodynamic Treatments

20.1 A teacher gives a child a piece of candy as a reward for answering a question correctly to encourage her students to participate more in class. This is an example of which of the following?

A. Classical conditioning.
B. Operant conditioning.
C. Behavioral activation.
D. Negative reinforcement.
E. Exposure.

The correct response is option B: Operant conditioning.

Operant conditioning involves changing behavior through administering positive or negative reinforcements (option B). Classical conditioning (option A) involves pairing two stimuli to elicit a target behavior in response to an unconditioned stimulus. Behavioral activation (option C) is a component of cognitive therapy that attempts to reengage patients in activities that they have stopped doing because of depression. Negative reinforcement (option D) decreases a target behavior rather than increasing it. Exposure involves putting patients in a feared situation in order to improve their coping ability (option E). **(pp. 521–522, 524)**

20.2 The candy in the previous question functions as which of the following?

A. Behavioral activation.
B. Negative reinforcement.
C. Conditioned stimulus.
D. Positive reinforcement.
E. Unconditioned stimulus.

The correct response is option D: Positive reinforcement.

The candy functions as positive reinforcement—a desirable stimulus is added to increase correct behavior (option D). Negative reinforcement (option B) involves avoiding or removing an undesirable stimulus in response to correct behavior. In this case, an example of negative reinforcement would be avoiding the humiliation of answering incorrectly. Conditioned and unconditioned stimuli (options C, E) are components of classical conditioning rather than operant conditioning. Behavioral activation (option A) is a component of cognitive therapy that attempts to reengage patients in activities that they have stopped doing because of depression. **(pp. 520–521, 524)**

20.3 An earthquake occurs during a psychopharmacology lecture, frightening several psychiatry residents, although it does not cause any serious damage. In the following weeks, attendance at the psychopharmacology lectures drops significantly. The psychopharmacology lecture functions as which of the following?

A. Conditioned stimulus.
B. Unconditioned stimulus.
C. Positive reinforcement.
D. Negative reinforcement.
E. Punishment.

The correct response is option A: Conditioned stimulus.

The psychopharmacology lecture works as the conditioned stimulus (option A). The residents learn to fear it through association because it is paired with the unconditioned stimulus of the earthquake (option B), which naturally causes fear. Positive reinforcement, negative reinforcement, and punishment (options C–E) are ways that behavior is modified through operant conditioning rather than classical conditioning. **(pp. 520–522)**

20.4   Gambling disorder develops through which of the following?

A. Classical conditioning.
B. Operant conditioning.
C. In vivo exposure.
D. Exposure.
E. Flooding.

The correct response is option B: Operant conditioning.

Gambling disorder develops through operant conditioning (option B). Winning functions as positive reinforcement given on a variable rather than fixed schedule. Classical conditioning (option A) involves learning to associate an unconditioned and a conditioned stimulus. In vivo exposure (option C) occurs when a patient engaging in behavior therapy is exposed to a real situation. Flooding (option E) involves teaching patients to extinguish anxiety produced by a feared stimulus through pacing them in continuous contact with the stimulus. Exposure (option D) involves placing patients in a situation they usually avoid in order to reduce the adaptive difficulties that are part and parcel of their psychiatric disorders. **(pp. 521–524)**

20.5   A therapist has a patient visualize being in an elevator to help him overcome his fear of elevators. This is an example of which of the following?

A. Relaxation training.
B. Imaginal exposure.
C. In vivo exposure.
D. Flooding.
E. Behavioral activation.

The correct response is option B: Imaginal exposure.

This is an example of imaginal exposure because the exposure to the feared situation—being in an elevator in this case—takes place within the imagination (option B). In vivo exposure (option C) is exposure to a real situation. Flooding (option D) involves teaching patients to extinguish anxiety produced by a feared stimulus through placing them in continuous contact with the stimulus and helping them learn that the stimulus does not in fact lead to any feared consequences. Relaxation training (option A) involves learning techniques such as deep breathing and progressive muscle relaxation to relieve anxiety. Behavioral activation (option E) is a component of behavioral therapy that attempts to reengage patients in activities that they have stopped doing because of depression. **(pp. 522–524)**

20.6   A therapist is working with a professional musician who is suffering from depression. The patient tells the therapist that she stopped playing the guitar 2 weeks ago because it no longer brings her pleasure. She previously had been playing the guitar for a few hours daily. The therapist proposes that she begin playing the guitar again every day, in spite of her lack of interest. This is an example of which of the following?

   A. Operant conditioning.
   B. Imaginal exposure.
   C. In vivo exposure.
   D. Flooding.
   E. Behavioral activation.

   The correct response is option E: Behavioral activation.

   This is an example of behavioral activation. The client is instructed to engage in her previous activities with the goal of restoring her functional status as part of treatment of her depression. Behavioral activation, which is also a component of cognitive therapy, seeks to reengage the patient in those activities, big and small, that lead to a rapid restoration of functioning. In turn, and consistent with behavioral theory, mood improves following restoration of important behavioral sequences in daily life, not the other way around. The other responses (options A–D) are components of behavior therapy. **(pp. 523–524)**

20.7   Which of the following is *not* part of Beck's cognitive triad of depression?

   A. Negative view of oneself.
   B. Negative view of relationships.
   C. Negative view of the future.
   D. Negative interpretation of experience.
   E. More than one of the above.

   The correct response is option B: Negative view of relationships.

Beck's cognitive triad of depression is a negative view of oneself, a negative view of the future, and a negative interpretation of experience (options A, C, D). Certainly, patients with depression often have a negative view of their relationships, but this is not a key part of Beck's cognitive triad (option B). **(p. 526)**

20.8 Learning to correct automatic thoughts, schemas, and distortions is a key part of which kind of therapy?

A. Behavioral therapy.
B. Cognitive-behavioral therapy.
C. Interpersonal therapy.
D. Psychodynamic psychotherapy.
E. Supportive psychotherapy.

The correct response is option B: Cognitive-behavioral therapy.

Learning to correct automatic thoughts, schemas, and distortions are integral to cognitive-behavioral therapy (option B). Behavioral therapy (option A) emphasizes correction of observable objective behavior rather than cognitions. Interpersonal therapy (option C) emphasizes improving interpersonal relationships by working on specific problem areas that may be interfering with self-esteem and interpersonal interactions. Psychodynamic therapy (option D) works on reviewing early and current relationships utilizing concepts derived from psychoanalysis, such as transference. Supportive psychotherapy (option E) involves providing affirmations and specific advice to help people cope with their stressors. **(pp. 520, 527, 531–533)**

20.9 An overzealous premedical student believes that she must get a perfect score on all of her assignments to have a chance of getting in to medical school lest she be forced to spend the rest of her career working in the food service industry. This is an example of which of the following?

A. Overgeneralization.
B. Selective abstraction.
C. Dichotomous thinking.
D. Personalization.
E. Magnification and minimization.

The correct response is option C: Dichotomous thinking.

Dichotomous thinking is a cognitive distortion in which the patient sees things in an all-or-none way (option C). The student in this example feels that she needs to have absolutely perfect marks or she will be a failure. Overgeneralization (option A) involves making general conclusions about overall experiences and relationships based on a single instance. Selective abstraction (option B) is taking a detail out of context and using it to denigrate the entire experience. Personalization (option D) is interpreting events as reflecting on oneself when they have no relation to the individual. Magnification and minimization (option E) involve altering the significance of specific events in a way that is structured by negative interpretations. (pp. 527–528)

20.10 A chess player wins three matches and loses one. He concludes that he got lucky in the three matches that he won and that he lost the other match because he is a terrible chess player. This is an example of which of the following?

A. Arbitrary inference.
B. Overgeneralization.
C. Dichotomous thinking.
D. Personalization.
E. Magnification and minimization.

The correct response is option E: Magnification and minimization.

The chess player is minimizing his successes, attributing them to luck, and magnifying his loss, taking it as evidence that he is a terrible player. This is magnification and minimization. (pp. 527–528)

20.11 A hard-working business woman arrives 30 minutes late to work because of an unexpected traffic jam caused by a car accident. She berates herself for her lack of responsibility and punctuality. This is an example of which of the following?

A. Arbitrary inference.
B. Overgeneralization.
C. Dichotomous thinking.
D. Personalization.
E. Magnification and minimization.

The correct response is option D: Personalization.

This is an example of personalization. The businesswoman blames herself for being late when she had no way to control the unexpected event. **(p. 527)**

20.12 Which of the following represents a major difference between classical psychoanalysis and psychodynamic psychotherapy?

A. The patient is expected to do the majority of the talking.
B. One is rooted in theories developed by Freud and his followers.
C. One of the major goals is to develop insight.
D. The frequency of treatment sessions differs.
E. The neutrality of the therapist.

The correct response is option D: The frequency of treatment sessions differs.

In classical psychoanalysis, the patient comes for session 4–5 times a week for 50 minutes/session for 2–3 years, whereas in psychodynamic therapy, sessions are usually once or twice a week for 2–5 years (option D). Options A–C and E are common to both forms of therapy. **(pp. 530–531)**

20.13 One of your patients is experiencing stress and anxiety that you attribute to coping with the new responsibilities that come with parenthood. Which type of psychotherapy would be especially suited to address this sort of problem?

A. Behavioral therapy.
B. Cognitive-behavioral therapy.
C. Psychodynamic psychotherapy.
D. Interpersonal therapy.
E. Supportive therapy.

The correct response is option D: Interpersonal therapy.

The patient is having trouble with making a role transition. Role transitions are a key domain of interpersonal therapy (option D). That said, the patient could benefit from the therapies in options A–C and E. **(pp. 532–533)**

20.14 Which of the following is *not* one of the four domains of interpersonal therapy?

A. Grief.
B. Interpersonal disputes.
C. Acceptance and commitment.
D. Role transitions.
E. Interpersonal deficits.

The correct response is option C: Acceptance and commitment.

Acceptance and commitment therapy is a form of therapy that targets emotional regulation (option C). Options A, B, D, and E represent the four key domains of interpersonal therapy. **(p. 533)**

20.15 A 26-year-old woman seeks treatment of her mood instability, difficult relationships, and self-harming behaviors. She is angry and irritable and says that prior therapists have not helped. She takes fluoxetine for her depression and anxiety, but it provides little symptomatic relief. She asks if there is something else you can do for her. Which of the following programs may be beneficial to her?

A. Dialectical behavior therapy (DBT).
B. Mentalization therapy.
C. Systems Training for Emotional Predictability and Problem Solving (STEPPS).
D. Schema-focused therapy (SFT).
E. All of the above.

The correct response option is E: All of the above.

The woman in the vignette appears to have borderline personality disorder, which is challenging to treat and responds poorly to medication. Fortunately, there are now several evidence-based programs developed specifically to treat people with this condition. Perhaps the best known is DBT (option A), a program that combines group and individual therapy. Developed by Marcia Linehan in the 1980s initially as a treatment for suicidal women, borderline personality disorder is viewed as a disorder of emotional dysregulation. The intensive 1-year program includes a mix of psychotherapeutic techniques as diverse as cognitive-behavioral therapy and mindfulness meditation derived from Buddhist practice. Options B, C, and D are all group therapies that have been developed for borderline patients. The main barrier to treatment is that these programs may not be available. **(pp. 535–536)**

20.16 You are seeing a 23-year-old man with schizophrenia in your office. The patient does not have any active positive symptoms of psychosis but is very awkward in interpersonal interactions and has difficulty with everyday tasks (e.g., maintaining appropriate hygiene). Which form of therapy would be beneficial in order to improve this patient's functional status?

A. Behavioral therapy.
B. Cognitive-behavioral therapy.
C. Psychodynamic psychotherapy.
D. Interpersonal therapy.
E. Social skills training.

The correct response is option E: Social skills training.

Social skills training is a specific type of psychotherapy that focuses primarily on developing abilities in relating to others and in coping with the demands of daily life, and it can substantially improve the quality of life of patients with severe mental illness such as schizophrenia (option E). Other forms of therapy (options A–D) may have some benefit for this patient, but social skills training is the modality that will best address the patient's identified deficits. **(pp. 538–539)**

CHAPTER 21

Psychopharmacology and Electroconvulsive Therapy

21.1 What was the world's first antipsychotic?

A. Haloperidol.
B. Thioridazine.
C. Fluphenazine.
D. Chlorpromazine.
E. Trifluoperazine.

The correct response is option D: Chlorpromazine.

Chlorpromazine was introduced in 1952 by the French psychiatrists Jean Delay and Pierre Deniker after it was recognized that the drug had powerful calming effects on agitated psychotic patients. The trade name of chlorpromazine is Thorazine, which is easily confused with thioridazine (option B), another first-generation antipsychotic. Options A, C, and E are other first-generation antipsychotic drugs. **(pp. 541–542)**

21.2 Compared with chlorpromazine, haloperidol

A. Has more anticholinergic side effects.
B. Is less sedating.
C. Causes fewer extrapyramidal side effects (EPS).
D. Is more likely to cause orthostatic hypotension.
E. Is associated with a much greater incidence of metabolic syndrome.

The correct response is option B: Is less sedating.

Haloperidol is less sedating than chlorpromazine (option B), is less likely to cause orthostatic hypotension (option D), has fewer anticholinergic side effects (option A), and is more likely to cause extrapyramidal symptoms (option C). Second-generation antipsychotics are more likely to induce a metabolic syndrome (option E). **(p. 542)**

21.3   The potency of conventional antipsychotic drugs correlates most closely with which of the following?

    A. Affinity for 5-hydroxytryptamine (serotonin) type 2 receptor (5-HT_{2A}) receptors.
    B. Anticholinergic activity.
    C. Antihistaminic activity.
    D. Dopamine D_2 receptor affinity.
    E. Norepinephrine receptor affinity.

The correct response is option D: Dopamine D_2 receptor affinity.

The potency of conventional antipsychotic drugs correlates with their ability to block endogenous dopamine at dopamine D_2 receptors (option D). Second-generation antipsychotics are weaker D_2 blockers, and they additionally block 5-HT_{2A} (option A). Central 5-HT_{2A} receptor antagonism is believed to broaden the therapeutic effect of the drug while reducing the incidence of EPS associated with D_2 antagonists. Second-generation agents also have significant anticholinergic and antihistaminic activity (options B, C). Antipsychotics have some activity on the norepinephrine system (option E), but it does not correlate with its therapeutic potency. **(pp. 542–545)**

21.4   As a general rule, most oral antipsychotics have a half-life of about

    A. 1 hour.
    B. 4 hours.
    C. 12 hours.
    D. 1 day.
    E. 5 days.

The correct response is option D: 1 day.

Nearly all antipsychotics have a half-life of 24 hours or longer and have active metabolites with longer half-lives. However, depot formulations have even longer half-lives and may take 3–6 months to reach steady state. **(p. 545)**

21.5 Which of the cytochrome P450 (CYP) enzymes is involved in the metabolism of antipsychotic medications?

A. 2D6.
B. 1A2.
C. 3A4.
D. 2D6, 1A2, and 3A4.
E. Metabolism does not occur because they are renally excreted.

The correct response is option D: 2D6, 1A2, and 3A4.

The majority of conventional antipsychotics are metabolized by the CYP enzyme subfamilies, including 2D6, 1A2, and 3A4. Because of genetic variation, 5%–10% of whites poorly metabolize medications through the CYP2D6 pathway, as do a significant proportion of African Americans. This can result in higher antipsychotic blood levels than anticipated in some patients. **(p. 545)**

21.6 You are following a 21-year-old man with schizophrenia on an inpatient psychiatric unit for 4 weeks. The patient continues to be floridly psychotic in spite of increasing doses of haloperidol, administered as oral tablets. His haloperidol blood level is 1 ng/mL. What does this suggest?

A. Psychotic symptoms are refractory to treatment with haloperidol.
B. The patient is a rapid metabolizer of haloperidol.
C. The patient is not swallowing the haloperidol tablets.
D. This blood level suggests laboratory error.
E. Haloperidol blood levels do not correlate with treatment response.

The correct response is option C: The patient is not swallowing the haloperidol tablets.

With haloperidol, optimal response appears to be associated with serum concentrations between 5–15 ng/mL (option E). Because the patient in this scenario has a blood level of 1 ng/mL and continues to show significant psychosis, it is likely that he is "cheeking" his medications and spitting them out (option C). Although laboratory error (option D) is possible, it is less likely than option C. Option A is not appropriate because with such a low blood level, the psychiatrist cannot conclude the patient's disorder is treatment refractory. There is no reason given in the vignette to suggest the patient is a rapid metabolizer (option B). **(pp. 545–546)**

21.7   You are following a 21-year-old man with schizophrenia on an inpatient psychiatric unit for 6 weeks. The patient continues to be floridly psychotic in spite of increasing doses of haloperidol, administered as oral tablets. His haloperidol blood level is 15 ng/mL. What does this suggest?

A. Psychotic symptoms are refractory to treatment with haloperidol.
B. The patient is a rapid metabolizer of haloperidol.
C. The patient is not swallowing the haloperidol tablets.
D. This suggests laboratory error.
E. Haloperidol blood levels do not correlate with treatment response.

The correct response is option A: Psychotic symptoms are refractory to treatment with haloperidol.

Many patients have a delayed response to medication, but it is worrisome that after 4 weeks, with therapeutic blood levels, that he has not had any improvement (option A). If the patient were not swallowing the tablets (option C), he would not have such a high blood level of haloperidol. Laboratory errors (option D) are always a possibility but not as likely an explanation as refractory response to treatment. There is no reason given in the vignette to suggest the patient is a rapid metabolizer (option B). Option E is not appropriate because haloperidol blood levels are known to correlate with treatment response. **(p. 546)**

21.8   How long is an adequate trial of an antipsychotic drug?

A. 4–6 days.
B. 4–6 weeks.
C. 2–3 months.
D. 6–8 months.
E. The duration of an adequate trial depends on the specific agent.

The correct response is option B: 4–6 weeks.

An adequate trial of an antipsychotic should be from 4 to 6 weeks for any agent. The trial can be extended if a patient shows partial response after this time interval, but a change of agent should be considered if the patient shows no response. **(p. 546)**

21.9   What is the primary reason that clozapine is a second-line choice for treating psychosis?

A. Because many patients have refractory schizophrenia, clozapine is always in short supply.
B. Because clozapine can cause significant weight gain.
C. Because clozapine does not work as well as other antipsychotics for treating refractory symptoms.
D. Clozapine frequently causes agranulocytosis, making it necessary for patients to have their white blood cell counts checked regularly.
E. Because it takes 3–6 months to reach steady state.

The correct response is option D: Clozapine frequently causes agranulocytosis, making it necessary for patients to have their white blood cell counts checked regularly.

Clozapine is a second-line agent for treating schizophrenia because it can cause agranulocytosis, so it is necessary for patients starting clozapine to have their white blood cell counts checked weekly (option D). Clozapine works better than other antipsychotics for treating refractory symptoms (option C), but it is not usually in short supply (option A). Clozapine can cause weight gain, but other antipsychotics can as well (option B). Clozapine reaches steady state as quickly as other orally administered antipsychotics (option E). Depot injection antipsychotics such as haloperidol decanoate can take 3–6 months to reach steady state. **(pp. 546, 549–550)**

21.10 You are seeing a 21-year-old man with schizophrenia in the outpatient clinic. His psychotic symptoms have been in remission on a moderate dose of haloperidol for the past 3 years. He has been admitted to the hospital three times for acute psychosis but has never engaged in dangerous behavior during episodes of acute psychosis. He is in school and reports that he has a good mood. The patient is interested in discontinuing antipsychotic medications, although he has tolerated the medication well. What is your recommendation?

A. "Now would be a good time for a trial without medications."
B. "We should make sure that you remain stable for another 2 years before attempting to discontinue medications."
C. "You should take the medication for the rest of your life."
D. "Let's try a new antipsychotic medication."
E. "Let's substitute a mild antidepressant for your other symptoms such as lack of motivation."

The correct response is option B: "We should make sure that you remain stable for another 2 years before attempting to discontinue medications."

About 75% of stable patients on antipsychotics will relapse within 6–24 months when taken off of their medications compared with 30% of those who continue to take medications. Following an initial episode of psychosis, patients should remain on medications for at least 1–2 years, whereas patients with multiple episodes should remain on medications for at least 5 years prior to attempting to discontinue medications. Patients with a history of becoming dangerous to themselves or others should remain on antipsychotics indefinitely. Some schizophrenic patients will benefit from antidepressants for an accompanying depression, which is not true for this man. **(pp. 148 [Chapter 5], 546–547)**

21.11 A patient with schizophrenia is admitted to an inpatient unit for acute psychosis, agitation, and violent ideation. He has had two recent (and similar admissions), and he readily admits to not taking prescribed aripiprazole tablets because he believes they are poisoned. His symptoms have responded well historically to antipsychotics that have been prescribed while he is hospitalized. Which of the following is the best long-term strategy for managing the patient's symptoms?

A. Switch to haloperidol decanoate.

B. Restart aripiprazole.

C. Switch to clozapine.

D. Switch to haloperidol.

E. Switch to risperidone.

The correct response is option A: Switch to haloperidol decanoate.

A long-acting injectable antipsychotic is the best strategy for addressing the patient's medication noncompliance. It is not likely that he will continue to take oral medications after discharge given his history. Haloperidol decanoate injections can be given monthly. **(p. 547)**

21.12 You are seeing a 35-year-old woman with schizoaffective disorder in the outpatient clinic. The patient's psychotic symptoms have been well controlled on fluphenazine for the past several years. In interview, she displays abnormal involuntary movements of her mouth and tongue of which she is not aware. This most likely represents which of the following?

A. Pseudoparkinsonism.

B. Akathisia.

C. Tardive dyskinesia.

D. Acute dystonic reaction.

E. Anticholinergic side effect.

The correct response is option C: Tardive dyskinesia.

Tardive dyskinesia refers to abnormal movements, usually of the mouth and tongue, that develop with long-term antipsychotic therapy (option C). Options A, B, D, and E refer to other side effects of antipsychotic medications. **(pp. 547–549)**

21.13 A 19-year-old man recently started on haloperidol for schizophrenia comes to the clinic as a walk-in requesting to be seen urgently. The patient paces in the waiting room, and in interview has trouble remaining seated in his chair and stands up frequently. He complains of severe anxiety. Which of the following best explains the patient's symptoms?

A. Akathisia.

B. New onset of generalized anxiety disorder.

C. Mania.

D. Acute dystonic reaction.

E. Tardive dyskinesia.

The correct response is option A: Akathisia.

Akathisia is the most common form of extrapyramidal side effects associated with antipsychotic drugs, particularly first-generation antipsychotics such as haloperidol (option A). It is characterized by subjective feelings of anxiety and tension and objective fidgetiness and agitation. Given the patient's diagnosis and that the symptoms developed shortly after a patient was started on an antipsychotic medication, new onset of generalized anxiety disorder (option B), mania (option C), and tardive dyskinesia (option E), which does not present in this fashion, are unlikely. An acute dystonic reaction (option D) involves sustained muscle contractions rather than acute severe anxiety. **(pp. 548–549)**

21.14 A 42-year-old woman presents to the emergency room complaining of muscle stiffness. Her neck is twisted to the left, and she reports that she cannot move it. She was discharged from the inpatient psychiatric unit a day earlier after receiving treatment for an acute psychosis, during which treatment with an antipsychotic agent was initiated. What is the best way to manage her symptoms?

A. Permanently discontinue the antipsychotic drug.

B. Switch to a new antipsychotic drug.

C. Administer benztropine or diphenhydramine intramuscularly.

D. Treatment with an oral benzodiazepine.

E. Psychotherapy for conversion disorder.

The correct response is option C: Administer benztropine or diphenhydramine intramuscularly.

The patient has an acute dystonic reaction as a side effect of an antipsychotic agent. This should respond to intramuscular benztropine or diphenhydramine within 20–30 minutes. Prophylactic benztropine may be given for the first 2 weeks of therapy with a conventional antipsychotic, but indefinite treatment with benztropine or a benzodiazepine is usually not necessary, because dystonic reactions tend not to recur. This patient has a medication side effect, not a conversion disorder, therefore psychotherapy is not indicated. **(p. 549)**

21.15 Which of the following is *not* an anticholinergic adverse effect of antipsychotics?

A. Diarrhea.
B. Urinary retention.
C. Blurry vision.
D. Dry mouth.
E. Exacerbation of narrow-angle glaucoma.

The correct response is option A: Diarrhea.

Constipation, not diarrhea, is an anticholinergic side effect of antipsychotics (option A). Options B–E are typical anticholinergic side effects that tend to commonly occur with low-potency agents such as chlorpromazine. **(p. 549)**

21.16 It has been recommended to regularly monitor body mass index (BMI), blood pressure, fasting glucose, and lipid panels for patients who are taking which of the following?

A. Haloperidol.
B. Risperidone.
C. Venlafaxine.
D. Sertraline.
E. Nortriptyline.

The correct response is option B: Risperidone.

Because second-generation antipsychotics (e.g., risperidone) are linked with metabolic abnormalities, it is recommended that patients have baseline measures of BMI, waist circumference, blood pressure, fasting glucose, and lipid panels (option B). Afterward, blood pressure, lipid panels, and fasting glucoses should be followed every 3 months, then annually. Options A and C–E are medications from other classes without standard guidelines for measuring these parameters. **(p. 550)**

21.17 A 45-year-old woman who takes haloperidol for her schizophrenia is admitted to a medical unit for rigidity, high fever, and mental status changes. Laboratory tests show elevated creatinine phosphokinase and liver enzymes. What is the most important aspect of acute care for this patient?

A. Start dantrolene.
B. Start bromocriptine.
C. Start electroconvulsive therapy (ECT).
D. Stop haloperidol and provide supportive care.
E. Transfer to psychiatric unit because this is a side effect of a psychotropic agent.

The correct response is option D: Stop haloperidol and provide supportive care.

Neuroleptic malignant syndrome (NMS) is a medical emergency. It develops as an adverse effect of antipsychotics, more commonly conventional antipsychotics such as haloperidol. The most important part of treatment is to stop the offending agent and provide supportive care (option D). Dantrolene and bromocriptine (options A, B) have been used to treat the condition, but there is no standardized treatment. ECT (option C) has been used for patients who do not improve with medical management. NMS should be managed on a medical unit rather than a psychiatric unit (option E). **(pp. 550–551)**

21.18 You are treating a 35-year-old man for a major depressive episode and narcissistic personality disorder. He demands that he receive the most effective antidepressant available. What do you do?

A. Prescribe levomilnacipran because it is one of the newest antidepressants.
B. Prescribe escitalopram, because it is a standard selective serotonin reuptake inhibitor (SSRI).
C. Prescribe venlafaxine because of its dual action in targeting norepinephrine and serotonin neurotransmission.
D. Advise him that, for the most part, all antidepressants are equally effective.
E. Recommend psychotherapy to address his underlying narcissism.

The correct response is option D: Advise him that, for the most part, all antidepressants are equally effective.

Generally speaking, antidepressants are equally effective, with 65%–70% response rate within 4–6 weeks versus 25%–40% for a placebo. **(p. 552)**

21.19 Which type of depression is expected to respond best to an antidepressant?

    A. Persistent depressive disorder (dysthymia).
    B. Atypical depression.
    C. Depression with comorbid hypochondriasis.
    D. Depression with comorbid somatic symptom disorder.
    E. Melancholic depression.

The correct response is option E: Melancholic depression.

Depressed patients with melancholic symptoms (e.g., diurnal variation, psychomotor agitation or retardation, terminal insomnia, pervasive anhedonia) may respond better to antidepressants than do other depressed patients. Atypical depression may preferentially respond to monoamine oxidase inhibitors (MAOIs). **(pp. 552, 557, 567)**

21.20 Which SSRI has the longest half-life?

    A. Fluoxetine.
    B. Sertraline.
    C. Citalopram.
    D. Escitalopram.
    E. Paroxetine.

The correct response is option A: Fluoxetine.

Fluoxetine has the longest half-life of 2–3 days, and its major metabolite, norfluoxetine, has a half-life of 4–16 days. The other SSRIs have half-lives ranging from 15 to 35 hours. **(p. 558)**

21.21 Which of the following is *not* a typical SSRI adverse effect?

    A. Loose bowel movements.
    B. Anxiety.
    C. Sexual dysfunction.
    D. Nausea.
    E. Orthostatic hypotension.

The correct response is option E: Orthostatic hypotension.

Options A–D are typical side effects of SSRIs with the exception of orthostatic hypotension (option E), which is more typically associated with tricyclic antidepressants and MAOIs. **(p. 558)**

21.22 You prescribe citalopram to a 28-year-old man for obsessive-compulsive disorder. At follow-up, he reports his symptoms have greatly improved, but he has developed delayed ejaculation that interferes with a new relationship. All of the following strategies have been used to address this condition *except*

A. Switch to bupropion.
B. Taking bupropion in addition to sertraline.
C. Taking cyproheptadine prior to sexual activity.
D. Taking lorazepam prior to sexual activity.
E. Taking sildenafil prior to sexual activity.

The correct response is option D: Taking lorazepam prior to sexual activity.

The development of an SSRI-induced sexual disorder creates a dilemma for the psychiatrist, particularly if the patient has responded well to the drug. The best option is to stop the offending drug, but this may not be desirable, particularly if the patient—as in this vignette—has obsessive-compulsive disorder, which responds preferentially to these agents. All of the strategies in options A–C and E have been used and may help, except for taking lorazepam (option D). Lorazepam can help with hyperstimulation caused by an SSRI or with the SSRI discontinuation syndrome **(p. 558)**

21.23 A 55-year-old woman is brought to the emergency room with an altered mental status, flushing, diaphoresis, and myoclonic jerks She was recently started on a third antidepressant agent for treatment-refractory depression. What is the most likely diagnosis?

A. Catatonia.
B. Serotonin syndrome.
C. NMS.
D. SSRI discontinuation syndrome.
E. Acute dystonic reaction.

The correct response is option B: Serotonin syndrome.

Serotonin syndrome presents with typical symptoms of lethargy, restlessness, mental confusion, flushing, diaphoresis, tremor, and myoclonic jerks (option B). Untreated it can progress to hyperthermia, hypertonicity, rhabdomyolysis, renal failure, and death. Patients who are concurrently taking two or more drugs that boost central nervous system serotonin levels are at higher risk. Co-administration of an MAOI and an SSRI can trigger serotonin syndrome. Symptoms of serotonin discontinuation syndrome include nausea, headache, vivid dreams, irritability, and dizziness (option D). NMS (option C) is more characterized by rigidity, high fever, and elevated creatine phosphokinase in a patient on an antipsychotic medication. Catatonia and acute dystonic reactions (options A, E) are not characterized by flushing, diaphoresis, or myoclonic jerks. **(pp. 550, 558–559)**

21.24 Which antidepressant is contraindicated for a 45-year-old man with epilepsy?

 A. Venlafaxine.
 B. Mirtazapine.
 C. Trazodone.
 D. Bupropion.
 E. Desvenlafaxine.

The correct response is option D: Bupropion.

Bupropion can cause seizures, particularly at dosages >450 mg/day. Thus, it is contraindicated in patients with a seizure disorder or an eating disorder, because patients with eating disorders may have a lower seizure threshold from electrolyte abnormalities. Seizure is the major risk of bupropion overdose. **(p. 561)**

21.25 Which of the following patients is a good candidate for a trial of duloxetine?

 A. A 37-year-old woman with a history of multiple recent overdose attempts.
 B. A 60-year-old man with chronic depression and alcoholism.
 C. A 20-year-old man with depression, posttraumatic stress disorder, and insomnia.

D. A 54-year-old woman with depression partially controlled by an MAOI.

E. A 48-year-old man with major depression and neuropathic pain from diabetes mellitus.

The correct response is option E: A 48-year-old man with major depression and neuropathic pain from diabetes mellitus.

Duloxetine has U.S. Food and Drug Administration (FDA)–approved indications for major depression, generalized anxiety disorder, diabetic neuropathic pain, and fibromyalgia (option E). It can be fatal in doses as low as 1,000 mg, so it should be avoided in patients at high risk for overdose (option A), and it can cause hepatotoxicity, so it should be avoided in patients who drink heavily (option B) or have liver disease. As with most antidepressants, it should not be mixed with an MAOI (option D) because of the risk of serotonin syndrome. Mirtazapine would be a better choice for a patient with major depression, posttraumatic stress disorder, and insomnia, because it can help with sleep (option C). **(pp. 561–562)**

21.26 Which of the following antidepressants is a good choice for a 30-year-old man with a first episode of melancholic depression with predominant features of insomnia and weight loss?

A. Citalopram.
B. Bupropion.
C. Duloxetine.
D. Mirtazapine.
E. Venlafaxine.

The correct response is option D: Mirtazapine.

The medications in options A–C and E would not be contraindicated for this patient; however, mirtazapine (option D) would be a particularly good choice because it can help with sleep disturbance and, as a side effect, it increases appetite, which can lead to weight gain. **(p. 562)**

21.27 Which of the following antidepressants is widely used to treat insomnia?

A. Venlafaxine.
B. Duloxetine.

C. Trazodone.
D. Phenelzine.
E. Sertraline.

The correct response is option C: Trazodone.

Trazodone is widely used to treat insomnia because it is very sedating. **(p. 563)**

21.28 A 35-year-old man with treatment refractory depression presents to the emergency room because of a prolonged painful erection. He has been taking multiple psychotropic medications to treat his disorder, including sertraline, bupropion, buspirone, trazodone, and lithium. Which medication was most likely to have caused his condition?

A. Sertraline.
B. Bupropion.
C. Buspirone.
D. Trazodone.
E. Lithium.

The correct response is option D: Trazodone.

Priapism, a prolonged painful erection, is an uncommon side effect of trazodone but can occur. Men who are prescribed trazodone should be warned about this potential side effect and should be instructed to seek immediate medical attention should it occur. **(p. 563)**

21.29 What is the mechanism of action of the new antidepressant vilazodone?

A. It is an SSRI.
B. It is a serotonin-norepinephrine reuptake inhibitor (SNRI).
C. It is a dopamine D_2 receptor antagonist.
D. It is a serotonin reuptake inhibitor and serotonin 1A (5-HT_{1A}) receptor partial agonist.
E. It blocks serotonin 2 receptors and weakly inhibits serotonin reuptake.

The correct response is option D: It is a serotonin reuptake inhibitor and serotonin 1A (5-HT_{1A}) receptor partial agonist.

Vilazodone is a serotonin reuptake inhibitor and 5-HT$_{1A}$ receptor partial agonist. Vilazodone is not a conventional SSRI or SNRI, and it does not block D$_2$ receptors. **(p. 564)**

21.30 Which of the following tricyclic antidepressants has an established therapeutic range?

    A. Amitriptyline.
    B. Nortriptyline.
    C. Doxepin.
    D. Clomipramine.
    E. Protriptyline.

The correct response is option B: Nortriptyline.

The therapeutic range of nortriptyline is 50–150 ng/mL. Desipramine and imipramine also have established therapeutic ranges. That said, there is no reason to routinely obtain plasma levels, particularly when the patient is doing well. Blood levels are helpful in cases of drug overdose and may also be useful when evaluating a patient's failure to respond adequately, significant symptoms of toxicity, or suspected noncompliance; in establishing a therapeutic window; and in setting dosage levels for a patient with significant cardiac or other medical disease (when it is desirable to keep the blood level at the lower range of the therapeutic value). **(p. 565)**

21.31 Why are MAOIs not more widely used to treat depression?

    A. Because of the required long washout period when transitioning a patient to or from an MAOI to avoid serotonin syndrome.
    B. Because when combined with foods that contain tyramine, a hypertensive crisis may result.
    C. Because they are potent α-adrenergic blockers and thus cause a high frequency of orthostatic hypotension.
    D. Because patients prescribed MAOIs need to carry a list of prohibited foods and wear a medical bracelet that indicates they are taking an MAOI and should carry a 10-mg tablet of nifedipine with them at all times.
    E. All of the above.

The correct response is option E: All of the above.

All of these are reasons that MAOIs are not commonly used. Although MAOIs may be helpful for cases of atypical depression, it is uncommon for such a patient to be started on an MAOI as a first choice. **(pp. 566–568)**

21.32 Which type of antidepressant should be used in a patient with a first episode of major depression?

A. Tricyclic antidepressant.
B. SSRI.
C. SNRI.
D. MAOI.
E. Any of the above.

The correct response is option B: SSRI.

All things being equal, treatment should begin with an SSRI because these medications are effective, well tolerated, and generally safe in overdose. **(p. 568)**

21.33 What is a reasonable length for an adequate trial of an antidepressant?

A. 3–5 days.
B. 3–5 weeks.
C. 1–2 months.
D. 3–4 months.
E. It depends on the agent.

The correct response is option C: 1–2 months.

Antidepressant trials should last 1–2 months. If a patient does not respond at 4 weeks on the target dosage, options to consider are increasing the dose or switching to a different antidepressant. **(p. 570)**

21.34 A 25-year-old man with a well-established diagnosis of bipolar disorder presents to the emergency room, having been brought in by the police for disruptive behavior. He has not been sleeping for the past 3 days, and he believes he is Jesus. He is very agitated, and you feel that he is potentially dangerous. Which medication should you give him in the emergency room?

A. Lithium.
B. Valproate.
C. Lamotrigine.
D. Haloperidol.
E. Carbamazepine.

The correct response is option D: Haloperidol.

Mood-stabilizing medications such as lithium or carbamazepine take 5–7 days to have a noticeable effect. The patient would benefit from prompt initiation of a mood stabilizer to treat his mania, but an antipsychotic such as haloperidol with or without a benzodiazepine would provide immediate sedation and tranquilization. **(pp. 546, 572)**

21.35 Which of the following medications has been shown to reduce suicidal behavior?

A. Valproate.
B. Lithium.
C. Carbamazepine.
D. Lamotrigine.
E. Alprazolam.

The correct response is option B: Lithium.

Lithium carbonate is one of the few drugs demonstrated to reduce suicidal behaviors, but care should be taken because lithium is more dangerous in overdose than an SSRI antidepressant. **(p. 572)**

21.36 Which of the following is *not* an appropriate use of lithium?

A. Prophylaxis of manic episodes in bipolar patients.
B. Reducing the severity of manic episodes.
C. Adjunctive treatment to prevent recurrences of depression in patients with unipolar major depression.
D. Achieving rapid sedation of an acutely agitated manic patient.
E. Prophylaxis of depressive episodes in bipolar patients.

The correct response is option D: Achieving rapid sedation of an acutely agitated manic patient.

Lithium is a remarkable drug that can prevent and moderate mood episodes in bipolar patients (options A, B, E) and can also help to prevent recurrence of depression in patients with unipolar depression (option C). It can be used to treat mood episodes in schizoaffective disorder. It is sometimes used to treat aggressive behavior, but an antipsychotic and/or benzodiazepine is best for rapid sedation of an agitated patient (option D). **(p. 572)**

21.37 When is the best time to check a lithium blood level?

A. 8 hours after the last dose for a manic patient and 18 hours after the last dose for a euthymic patient.
B. 12 hours after the last dose.
C. 8 hours after the last dose.
D. 18 hours after the last dose.
E. Accurate lithium levels can be obtained at any time because the elimination half-life of lithium is 36 hours.

The correct response is option B: 12 hours after the last dose.

Lithium levels should be checked 12 hours after the last dose. Manic patients clear lithium more quickly than euthymic patients because they are overly active and have a higher glomerular filtration rate, but the standard rule is to check the level 12 hours after the last dose whether the patient is manic, euthymic, or depressed. **(pp. 572–573)**

21.38 Which mood-stabilizing agent does *not* undergo mostly hepatic metabolism?

A. Valproate.
B. Lamotrigine.
C. Lithium.
D. Carbamazepine.
E. Aripiprazole.

The correct response is option C: Lithium.

Lithium is not metabolized and is renally excreted (option C). Options A, B, D, and E all undergo hepatic metabolism. **(pp. 545, 572–573)**

21.39 Which mood-stabilizing agent can in rare cases cause Stevens-Johnson syndrome?

A. Valproate.
B. Lamotrigine.
C. Lithium.
D. Carbamazepine.
E. Aripiprazole.

The correct response is option B: Lamotrigine.

In rare cases, lamotrigine can cause the potentially life-threatening Stevens-Johnson syndrome and toxic epidermal necrolysis. It should not be mixed with valproate, because combination therapy increases the risk. **(pp. 577–578)**

21.40 For which of the following cases is lamotrigine monotherapy most appropriate?

A. A patient with bipolar I disorder and a history of multiple hospitalizations for mania and a history of nonresponse to lithium.
B. A patient with bipolar I disorder with a history of multiple hospitalizations for mania and a history of response to lithium.
C. A patient with bipolar I disorder who presents with irritable mania.
D. A patient with bipolar disorder with mixed mania and depression.
E. A patient with bipolar I disorder with several severe depressive episodes and infrequent manic episodes.

The correct response is option E: A patient with bipolar I disorder with several severe depressive episodes and infrequent manic episodes.

Lamotrigine appears to be most effective in delaying the time to occurrence of depressive episodes and may be effective in the treatment of acute depressive episodes as well (option E). Patients with multiple hospitalizations for mania and a history of nonresponse to lithium (option A), patients with irritable mania (option C), and patients in a mixed episode (option D) would be good candidates for valproate. Patients with multiple hospitalizations for mania and a history of response to lithium (option B) are good candidates for lithium. **(pp. 575, 577–578)**

21.41 Which patient with bipolar disorder is a good candidate for carbamazepine therapy?

A. A patient with irritable mania who has not responded to lithium.
B. A patient in a mixed episode.
C. A patient with more than four mood episodes per year who has not responded to lithium.
D. A patient with mostly depressed episodes and mild infrequent hypomanic episodes.
E. None of the above.

The correct response is option C: A patient with more than four mood episodes per year who has not responded to lithium.

Carbamazepine may be more effective in patients who cycle rapidly (meaning patients who have more than four mood episodes per year) and who do not respond to lithium. Patients with irritable mania or mixed episodes may respond better to valproate. Lamotrigine would be a good choice for a patient with mostly depressive episodes and mild infrequent hypomanic episodes. **(pp. 575–577)**

21.42 Which neurotransmitter is intimately involved in the mechanism of action for benzodiazepines?

A. Glutamate.
B. Norepinephrine.
C. Gabapentin.
D. γ-Aminobutyric acid (GABA).
E. Serotonin.

The best response is option D: γ-Aminobutyric acid (GABA).

Benzodiazepines are believed to exert their effects by binding to specific benzodiazepine receptors in the brain. The receptors are intimately linked to receptors for GABA, a major inhibitory neurotransmitter. By binding to benzodiazepine receptors, the drugs potentiate the actions of GABA, leading to a direct anxiolytic effect on the limbic system. Gabapentin, of course, is a drug and not a neurotransmitter. **(p. 579)**

21.43 Benzodiazepines are remarkably versatile drugs. These medications used to treat all of the following *except*

A. Seizure disorders.
B. Anxiety.
C. Alcohol withdrawal.
D. Sleep disorders.
E. Major depression.

The correct response is option E: Major depression.

Benzodiazepines are useful for the treatment of generalized anxiety disorder, especially when severe. Many patients benefit when their anxiety is acute and problematic; these drugs generally should be given for short periods (e.g., weeks or months). Patients with mild anxiety may not need medication and can be successfully managed with behavioral interventions (e.g., progressive muscle relaxation). These drugs may be useful in treating depression, but they have no demonstrated antidepressant effect, and their use is mainly in treating those with an anxious form of depression. **(pp. 579–580)**

21.44 Which of the following medications has an FDA indication for the treatment of generalized anxiety disorder?

A. Buspirone.
B. Bupropion.
C. Alprazolam.
D. Aripiprazole.
E. None of the above.

The correct response option is A: Buspirone.

Buspirone has an FDA-approved indication for the treatment of generalized anxiety disorder (option A). The antidepressant bupropion (option B) has no role in treating anxiety, whereas aripiprazole (option D) is used to treat psychoses. Alprazolam (option C) has an indication to treat panic disorder but is not recommended to treat generalized anxiety disorder, except perhaps on a short-term basis as with the other benzodiazepines. **(pp. 579, 582)**

21.45 Extrapyramidal syndromes have been treated with all of the following medications *except*

A. Propranolol.
B. Diphenhydramine.
C. Amantadine.
D. Benztropine.
E. Trazodone.

The correct response is option E: Trazodone.

The choice of drug depends on the syndrome. Pseudoparkinsonism can be treated with benztropine or amantadine (options C, D). An acute dystonic reaction can be treated with intramuscular diphenhydramine (option B). Akathisias can be treated with propranolol (option A). Trazodone (option E) is not used to treat any of these syndromes. **(pp. 583–585)**

21.46 Which of the following conditions represents an absolute contraindication to administering ECT?

A. Recent myocardial infarction.
B. Unstable coronary artery disease.
C. Space-occupying brain lesions.
D. Venous thrombosis.
E. Chronically low platelet count.

The correct response is option C: Space-occupying brain lesions.

Relative contraindications include recent (i.e., within 1 month) myocardial infarction (option A), unstable coronary artery disease (option B), uncompensated congestive heart failure, uncontrolled hypertensive cardiovascular disease, venous thrombosis (option D), and chronically low platelet count (option E). Space-occupying brain lesions and other causes of increased intracranial pressure, such as recent intracerebral hemorrhage, unstable aneurysms, or vascular malformations are the only absolute contraindications to ECT (option C). **(p. 587)**

21.47 A 36-year-old woman is receiving ECT for treatment of her major depression. What should she be told about possible adverse effects of the treatment?

A. She may have permanent memory loss that will be most dense around the time of treatment.
B. She will have no memory loss because the psychiatrist will use unilateral lead placement.
C. She will have permanent memory loss that will mainly involve new memories following the conclusion of the treatment.
D. She will have no memory loss because the psychiatrist will use the minimal amount of electricity needed to be therapeutic.
E. None of the above.

The correct response is option A: She may have permanent memory loss that will be most dense around the time of treatment.

The most troublesome long-term effect of ECT is memory loss. Because ECT disrupts new memories that have not been incorporated into long-term memory stores, ECT can cause anterograde and retrograde amnesia that is most dense around the time of treatment. The anterograde component usually clears quickly, but the retrograde amnesia can extend back to months before treatment. Not all patients experience memory loss, and unilateral electrode placement, modification of the pulse wave, and the use of low dosages of electricity help minimize any loss that occurs. They do not prevent memory loss from occurring, however. Patients must be told that permanent memory loss can occur. **(p. 589)**

CPSIA information can be obtained
at www.ICGtesting.com
Printed in the USA
LVOW04s0801150316
479144LV00002B/2/P